RISK, CHANCE, AND CAUSATION

Risk, Chance, and Causation

Investigating the Origins and
Treatment of Disease

MICHAEL B. BRACKEN

Yale
UNIVERSITY PRESS
NEW HAVEN AND LONDON

Published with assistance from the foundation established in memory of
Philip Hamilton McMillan of the Class of 1894, Yale College.

Yale University Press books may be purchased in quantity for educational, business,
or promotional use. For information, please e-mail sales.press@yale.edu (U.S. office)
or sales@yaleup.co.uk (U.K. office).

Set in Electra type by Newgen North America.
Printed in the United States of America.

Library of Congress Cataloging-in-Publication Data
Bracken, Michael B., 1942–
Risk, chance, and causation : investigating the origins and treatment
of disease / Michael B. Bracken.
p. ; cm.
Includes bibliographical references and index.
ISBN 978-0-300-18884-4 (cloth : alk. paper)
I. Title.
[DNLM: 1. Disease–etiology.   2. Risk Factors.   3. Therapeutics. QZ 40]
616.07′1—dc23
2012045173

A catalogue record for this book is available from the British Library.

This paper meets the requirements of ANSI/NISO Z39.48-1992
(Permanence of Paper).

10 9 8 7 6 5 4 3 2 1

To
Kai, Lucian, Lilén, and Finn
I am not so sanguine as to believe that when you are able
to read this book, its lessons will have been learned:
plus ça change, plus c'est la même chose.

CONTENTS

CONTENTS

ACKNOWLEDGMENTS

Many people over a lifetime of work have helped form the ideas and concepts explored in this book. They are far too many to name, but I hope they will recognize their contributions and forgive me for not mentioning them individually. For the book itself, I am grateful to Yale University for the sabbatical that allowed me to complete the project and to the Fellows of Green Templeton College at Oxford University for providing an academic home away from home for many years. Lia Kidd has kept my professional life in good order for more years than we both care to remember, and she solved numerous technical problems during the production of the manuscript and proofread the entire book more than once. Others at the Yale Center for Perinatal, Pediatric, and Environmental Epidemiology assisted in obtaining copyrights and TIFFs and greatly helped in the book's production: thank you Geetanjoli Banerjee, Susan Chase Jones, Jodi O'Sullivan and Matt Wilcox. At Yale University Press, Sara Hoover and Jean Thomson Black, my editor, have been supportive throughout the project. I especially appreciate the thoughtful and sensitive approach to copy editing by Eliza Childs. Iain Chalmers is a lifetime supporter and collaborator, and I am grateful to him for reading the chapter that relates to his work. Andrew De-Wan, Ted Holford, and Jessica Illuzzi are all valued colleagues, and they made helpful comments on chapters in their specialties. Students in my "Evidence-Based Medicine and Health Care" course at Yale have never failed to provide critical feedback, and their reading of various chapters is equally appreciated. Emmanuelle Delmas-Glass was the perfect foil for me to bounce ideas off as she has all the qualities of the book's intended audience—bright people without any particular professional interest in the topic. My wife Maryann, as always, rose to the challenge and was a keen editor and enthusiastic supporter of this work. Of course, any errors and all the strong opinions are entirely my own.

ABBREVIATIONS

μg	Microgram
A	Adenine
ACS	American Cancer Society
AD	Alzheimer's disease
AIDS	Acquired immune deficiency syndrome
AMD	Adult macular degeneration
ARRIVE	Animal research: reporting in vivo experiments
ASD	Autism spectrum disorder
BBC	British Broadcasting Corporation
BCE	Before the Common Era
BCS	Breast conserving surgery
BID	Bis in die (twice a day)
BL-4	Biosafety Level 4 (facility)
BP	British Petroleum
BPA	Bisphenol-A
BPD	Bronchopulmonary dysplasia
BSE	Breast self-examination
C	Cytosine
CA-125	Cancer antigen 125
CAST	Chinese Acute Stroke Trial
CDC	Centers for Disease Control and Prevention
CE	Common Era

CI	Confidence interval
CNS	Central nervous system
CNV	Copy number variation
CRASH	Corticosteroid Randomization after Severe Head (injury)
DDT	Dichlorodiphenyltrichloroethane
DES	Diethylstilbestrol
DNA	Deoxyribonucleic acid
E	Expected number of events
EMF	Electromagnetic fields
EPA	Environmental Protection Agency
F	Fahrenheit
FDA	Food and Drug Administration
G	Guanine
g	Gram
GI	Gastrointestinal
GPS	Global Positioning System
GWAS	Genome-wide association studies
HIV	Human immunodeficiency virus
HMS	Her Majesty's Ship
HPV	Human papilloma virus
HRT	Hormone replacement therapy
HuGENet	Human Genome Epidemiology Network
HupA	Huperzine A
IARC	International Agency for Research on Cancer
IOM	Institute of Medicine
IPDMA	Individual patient data meta-analysis
IQ	Intelligence quotient
IRBs	Institutional Review Boards
ISIS2	Second International Study of Infarct Survival
IST	International Stroke Trial
IVF	In vitro fertilization
JAMA	*Journal of the American Medical Association*
LDL	Low-density lipoprotein
ml	Milliliter

MMR	Measles-mumps-rubella
mRNA	Messenger ribonucleic acid
NAS	National Academy of Science
NICU	Newborn intensive care unit
NIH	National Institutes of Health
NNH	Number Needed to Harm
NNT	Number Needed to Treat
O	Observed events
ODPT	Oxford Database of Perinatal Trials
OR	Odds Ratio
PAH	Polycyclic aromatic hydrocarbon
PFC	Perfluorinated compound
PM	Particulate matter
PSA	Prostate-specific antigen
RCT	Randomized Controlled Trial
RD	Risk Difference
RNA	Ribonucleic acid
RR	Relative risk or risk ratio
RVOTO	Right ventricular outflow tract obstructive (defect)
SIDS	Sudden infant death syndrome
SNP	Single nucleotide polymorphism
SSRIs	Selective serotonin re-uptake inhibitors
T	Thymine
TNFA	Tumor necrosis factor gene
tPA	Tissue plasminogen activator
VIGOR	Vioxx Gastrointestinal Outcomes Research
WHO	World Health Organization

ONE

Risk, Chance, and Causation

Investigating the Origins and Treatment of Disease

> Oh Lord, you did not give us enough evidence.
> —*Bertrand Russell*

> Bliss in proof—and proved a very woe.
> —*William Shakespeare, Sonnet 129*

Bertrand Russell was, of course, referring to God's existence when he decried a lack of evidence, but he might just as well have been referring to the absence of reliable evidence pertaining to risk in many aspects of everyday life and the difficulty that scientists have in producing reliable estimates of risk or, indeed, assessing whether there is any risk at all. How do scientists attempt to separate chance associations, the links between environmental agents and disease, from real ones? And how is an association, once demonstrated, determined to be causal? The public is bombarded on a daily basis by claims that this food supplement is essential for health or that chemical is hazardous, that medicines thought initially to be beneficial are now dangerous, or that some nutritional element will extend life, cause cancer, or improve or worsen our chance of senile dementia. It is not surprising that there is confusion, because the science of determining risk and causality is itself uncertain. The science most responsible for examining whether humans are likely to benefit or be at risk from environmental exposure, or whether medicines are effective and safe, is epidemiology, and epidemiologists themselves do not completely agree how to evaluate risk.

There are only vaguely agreed-upon criteria for when causation has been demonstrated. It is patently obvious that many published studies must be wrong because they completely contradict other studies, and all of them cannot be correct. Studies of risk are plagued with numerous biases—some avoidable but others not—and the publication process for scientific papers guarantees that many incorrect studies will be published. This book explores the reasons why it is so difficult to reliably assess individual and public exposure to risk. It offers recommendations for improving the scientific methods, the publication process, and synthesis of risk studies, and it suggests how research on risk should be interpreted by nonscientists.

The stakes are very high. For example, in 2002 a very large randomized trial[1] by the Women's Health Initiative[2] reported that women who used hor-

---

Box 1.1 Science and Journalism: An Uncertain Alliance.

Some journalists appear to be incensed by the failure of epidemiologists to provide replicable and consistent evidence as to the true risks or benefits of environmental and lifestyle exposures. Gary Taubes, writing in the journal *Science* in 1995, suggested that epidemiology had reached its limits and that "the search for subtle links between diet, lifestyle, or environmental factors and disease is an unending source of fear but often yields little certainty."[*] This statement provoked much commentary among epidemiologists, a lot of it very defensive, but led to little change. Other commentators were even more critical: "Closing down most university departments of epidemiology could extinguish both this endlessly fertile source of anxiety mongering while simultaneously releasing funds for serious research."[†]

A more realistic perspective was shown by Nicholas Wade, writing in the *New York Times:* "Journals like Science and Nature do not, and cannot, publish scientific truths. They publish roughly screened scientific claims which may or may not turn out to be true."[‡] We will see in this book why many studies of causation and health effects do indeed turn out not to be true.

[*]Taubes G. Epidemiology faces its limits. *Science.* 1995;269:164–169.
[†]Le Fanu J. *The rise and fall of modern medicine.* London: Little, Brown, 1999.
[‡]Wade N. Lowering expectations at science's frontier. *New York Times.* January 15, 2006.

mone replacement therapy (HRT) were at a 29 percent increased risk of cardiovascular heart disease. This conclusion was in direct contrast to earlier reports from large epidemiological studies of thousands of nurses that HRT protected against heart disease (a 39 percent *reduction* in risk in the major studies). It has also been reported from the Women's Health Initiative that breast cancer risk is increased by 24 percent in women using estrogen plus progestin, the most popular form of HRT therapy. During the decade since the first studies reporting benefit there was a substantial increase in the number of women using some form of HRT, following major promotion campaigns by industry and some medical professionals, so that 20 to 40 percent of all postmenopausal women in the United States eventually used HRT. After reports of the Women's Health Initiative trial were published, millions of women who had been on HRT therapy discontinued it, some with substantial difficulty.

The Women's Health Initiative trials have also shown that calcium and vitamin D supplementation do not protect against fractures in older women, and that low-fat diets do not lower the risk of invasive breast cancer, colorectal cancer, or heart disease.[3] Other large studies report that antioxidant supplementation increases, rather than as originally thought decreases, mortality,[4] that treatment with B vitamins did not lower the risk of second heart attack, as anticipated, but may instead be harmful.[5] These examples and many more will be discussed in later chapters.

Prompted by widespread marketing, millions of people use food supplements on a daily basis, expecting benefits to physical strength, agility, mental acuity, virility, and longevity. But what is the evidence that these pills and potions are beneficial? How do we know they do not cause harm? In most cases, there is none or at best limited scientific evidence to support the claims of effectiveness and no reassuring data about safety. At the same time, the medical profession treats patients with a wide variety of medications that have been approved by regulatory agencies (unless they are very old remedies and were grandfathered approval when the regulatory laws were first enacted) but about which doubts of safety subsequently arise. There is increasing use of what is an oxymoronic term: "alternative medical therapy" (if it is being administered to patients and is successful, why is it "alternate"; if it is not successful, it should not be part of medical therapy). We are also being increasingly screened, scanned, and imaged by a massive and vested corporate infrastructure, which rarely evaluates its technologies in a scientifically valid way, and for conditions that often remain untreatable or for which the available therapies have only marginal if any benefit.

The need for rigorous comparison of medical therapies to ascertain their effectiveness and safety, while now generally accepted by the medical and health professions, has only recently permeated the halls of the US Congress and the White House. Perhaps feeling the need to appear to be doing something novel, the term "comparative effectiveness" was coined in 2009 to describe the allocation of over one billion dollars to compare treatments for drugs, medical devices, surgery, and other ways of treating medical conditions. As we shall see, comparing the effectiveness of therapies is only one aspect of the evidence-based medicine paradigm (not least, safety is of equal interest), but what's in a name? Researchers welcomed this infusion of funds, a tiny percentage of the total US health care expenditures of $2.7 trillion in 2007, for testing rational therapies.

A Classic Example of Demonstrating Causality: Joseph Goldberger Studies Pellagra

It is instructive to begin our examination of risk, chance, and causation using a case example from the early years of epidemiology. Epidemiologists usually refer to John Snow's investigation of the cholera epidemics in nineteenth-century London as a classic example for documenting the cause of a disease, but as exemplary as this was, it was based entirely on observation; there was no experiment. We will discuss some of the key elements in Snow's work later in the book. Cholera is not the only early example of documenting the causes of infectious disease: smallpox, yellow fever, poliomyelitis, malaria, and in the recent past the identification of HIV as the cause of AIDS are all classic examples of inferring causality using traditional epidemiologic methods.

The work of Joseph Goldberger in early twentieth-century South Carolina provides an even more interesting example for our purposes because

it combines both an observational and an experimental approach to understanding the cause of pellagra. As observation and experiment are the two
pillars of modern epidemiological investigation, Goldberger's work remains
a classic in the annals of epidemiological investigation, although it is often
forgotten among the praise lauded on John Snow. Whereas almost all the
early studies of causation were of infectious or communicable disease, Goldberger was investigating a non-communicable disease, although he didn't
know it as he began his work. These diseases, the focus of much attention
at the present time, pose particular difficulties in assigning causation, and
this is what is of primary concern in this book. The attention to diet in the
pellagra research also presages a common current concern of broad public
interest: how much does our diet influence the risk of disease? It might be
argued that much of present-day diet supplement research would benefit
from following the precepts laid down by Goldberger.

Pellagra is a disease producing exfoliation of the skin not unlike leprosy,
digestive disorders, severe spinal pain, convulsions, depression, and severe
mental retardation. Despite these major symptoms, it was not recognized
as a distinct condition until late in the nineteenth century, and the first
estimates of incidence were reported in 1912, with 25,000 cases in the previous five years and a case fatality rate of 40 percent. The dominant causal
agent was thought to be an intestinal infection, susceptibility to which was
increased by a diet deficient in animal protein. In asking Goldberger to
investigate the cause of pellagra, the Surgeon General of the United States
called it "undoubtedly one of the knottiest and most urgent problems facing
the [public health] Service at the present time."[6]

In a brief report in 1914, Goldberger recognized that at the South Carolina State Hospital for the Insane, which recorded 98 deaths from pellagra
between 1909 and 1913, no deaths had occurred in nurses and attendants
who lived in very close proximity to the inmates and, indeed, among whom
there had been no cases of any kind.[7] Goldberger observed, "If pellagra be a
communicable disease, why should there be an exemption of the nurses and
attendants?" He went on to note that the diets of the nurses were more varied than those of the inmates and were supplemented by outside meals. He
also noted that pellagra is essentially a disease associated with rural poverty

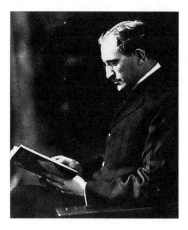

Figure 1.1. Joseph Goldberger, 1874–1929. Courtesy of the
Office of History, National Institutes of Health.

and that the diets of the rural poor were deficient in dairy produce and fresh
meat but had an excess of cereals. Only three months later, Goldberger,
writing to the Surgeon General, clearly specified the nutritional hypothesis:
"Evidence seems to be accumulating to show that pellagra is due to the use
of a dietary [*sic*] in which some essential element is reduced in amount or
from which it is altogether absent, or to the use of a dietary in which some
element is present in injurious amount."[8] At this stage, it remained uncertain whether the disease was from a deficiency or an excess of an unknown
constituent in the diet.

The next step in the investigation took place in two orphanages in Jack-
son, Mississippi, where the diet was supplemented with eggs, milk, legumes,
and meat, with reductions in corn, but the sanitary and hygienic conditions
were left unchanged. Among 67 pellagra patients at one orphanage, no recurrence of the disease was seen after the diet change, and none of the 99
non-pellagra patients at the start of the study contracted pellagra during the
new diet period. In the second orphanage, only one of 105 cases of pellagra
showed a recurrence, and 69 non-pellagra patients at the start of the new diet
continued to be free of disease. Similar results were reported from a Georgia
asylum where two wards were studied with almost identical dietary changes
to those in the orphanages. In the orphanage studies, the expected recur-

rence rates of disease could be predicted from earlier experience in the institution (they were 58 to 76 percent) and from other wards in the asylum not in the study (47 percent). The absence of any recurrence of pellagra in the patients with a supplemented diet provided powerful evidence in support of some aspect of diet as the source of the diseases. However, Goldberger was aware that some infectious disease, such as beriberi, could show changes in symptoms depending on the diet; moreover, the dietary changes were broad and did not permit any conclusions about specific nutrient sources. Goldberger's conclusions from the study were carefully circumscribed; he concluded that pellagra could be prevented by careful diet, but it is apparent that he is referring to the symptoms of the disease and not its underlying cause, the determination of which would require more research.[9]

At this stage in his investigations, Goldberger adopted an experimental approach, primarily to address the alternative explanation of the beriberi phenomenon, that diet might be influencing symptoms from an infection-caused disease. He used methods that would be considered highly unethical by modern researchers as the subjects were a dozen healthy prisoners, promised a pardon by the governor on completion of their participation in the study, who were fed a largely cereal diet thought to be responsible for inducing pellagra.[10]

The Rankin farm of the Mississippi State Penitentiary was the site of Goldberger's new study. Only white male convicts were given the opportunity to join, it is said, because they were least susceptible to the disease, and the 12 chosen lived in special quarters during the course of the study, which was to last for six months. The control group was the remaining farm convicts and staff. Of the 12 study subjects, one escaped and was replaced by another convict from the control group; a second developed prostatitis and was released from the experimental group and prison. With respect to hygiene, the convict controls were described as living in "dirty and vermin infested" quarters whereas the quarters of the "Pellagra Squad" were "regularly and thoroughly cleaned."

The diets of the study groups are described in great detail and offer an insight into the quality of meals served to convicts in that era. Over a six-month period, the most common components of the diet for the convict controls were cane "sirup" (585 servings) and biscuits (559 servings) with one serving each of fresh fish, ice cream, bean soup, and bananas, or assessed another way, 234 pounds of biscuit and 3 pounds of butter per person during the six months. The diet of the experimental subjects was deliberately altered in the following respects: fat and carbohydrate intake was similar but protein consumption reduced by a half and none of it was from animal sources. Milk, butter, peas, and beans were in the control diet but not the experimental group. The report also offers great detail into how many times the volunteer men were scrubbed and changed their underwear, reflecting an interest in other disease risk factors.

The results of the experiment were as hoped: 6 of the 11 volunteers developed what was described as evidence of pellagra as diagnosed by a panel of expert consultants but none of the much larger number of controls developed symptoms.[11] Goldberger and his colleagues were able to conclude that this experiment ruled out the infection hypothesis (the Pellagra Squad lived in much more hygienic conditions than the control convicts but still became ill) and clearly pointed to a dietary origin; moreover, it indicated some deficiency rather than an excessive amount of a dietary component. As far as the component of the diet itself, the study seemed to suggest a deficiency in protein and likely in an amino acid, but more detailed analysis was not possible from this study. More research was needed.[12]

At the same time that he was conducting his experiment in convicts, Goldberger reported a study where he and 15 other medical officers, showing remarkable fortitude, tried to inoculate themselves with a variety of material from pellagra cases, specifically "blood, nasopharyngeal secretions, epidermal scales from pellagrous skin lesions, urine and feces. The blood was administered by intramuscular or subcutaneous injection, the secretions by application to the mucosa of the nose and nasopharynx, scales and excreta by mouth."[13] Moreover, the inoculations were repeated several times. None of the subjects showed any symptoms of pellagra. Goldberger stoically remarked, "When one considers the relatively enormous quantities of filth taken the reactions were surprisingly slight." There followed a series of studies looking at the prevalence of pellagra in relation to the cost of food, more investigations of diet, examination of other risk factors, particularly gender, age, season, and occupation, more detailed examination of sanitary factors (water and sewage supplies), income, and a study of villages where pellagra seemed to be especially endemic.[14]

After this series of classic epidemiological studies, many of which would be typical of modern disease investigation, Goldberger started to focus on the causative agent itself, which he had deduced was likely to be an amino acid deficiency. In a series of relatively small studies, pellagra cases were each supplemented with elements of the diet found helpful in the orphanage studies, specifically: dried soy beans, casein, dried milk, and brewers' yeast. While some patients in the first three treatments developed pellagra, none of the 26 patients administered brewers' yeast did, although it was expected that 40 to 50 percent would relapse.[15] Subsequent work in the laboratory with a variety of animals suggested to Goldberger that what he called P-P, the active "pellagra-prevention" agent, was a factor in vitamin B. Goldberger died in 1929 before he was able to further identify P-P, but later work by various scientists showed that P-P was nicotinic acid, a product of the amino acid tryptophan.

I have labored through Goldberger's work because it represents a seminal contribution to understanding the causality of what was in his time a serious and not uncommon condition, using methods that, while technically less sophisticated than would be used by a scientist today, represent a modern conceptual framework (excepting, happily, the self-inoculation with "filth"). Classic risk factor epidemiology was adequate to strongly support the hypothesis for a dietary association, and experiments where dietary change was used both to prevent the disease and to induce it were crucial to showing causation. When needed, Goldberger combined observational studies with experimental work to test crucial hypotheses about the disease. Different disease rates were not statistically analyzed, which was not unusual in the science journals of that period, but they clearly met what is now mischievously known as the "intra-ocular impact test"—that is, it hits you "between the eyes" that there was a substantial reduction in the pellagra rate after the improved diet was instituted. Modern epidemiologists would be ecstatic if their studies showed similarly strong results. Further experiments by other scientists refined the diet and identified the actual nutrient whose deficiency caused pellagra. One has to feel that only Goldberger's premature death stopped him from getting there himself.

Modern Epidemic Investigation: A Global Endeavor

The investigation of pellagra used both observational and experimental methods to look for a cause, but that is where the similarities part company with modern epidemic investigation. Now the race to find a cause, a vaccine, and a cure is fast paced and furious. Viewers of Steven Soderbergh's 2011 film *Contagion* were offered a surprisingly accurate accounting of the process. Many modern epidemics are the result of (and most certainly will continue to be so) newly mutated viruses emerging from Africa and Asia where humans live in close proximity to animals. In *Contagion,* the virus was the product of a bat and pig virus genetically changed so that DNA from each species was combined with DNA from a human virus making it transmissible from one person to another. Soderbergh cleverly starts his film on day two of the epidemic when the first case, Beth, played by an infected Gwyneth Paltrow, passes the virus on to hundreds of contacts while traveling from Hong Kong to Chicago and then Minneapolis. The virus spreads around the world at an exponential rate causing mayhem and huge social upheaval. Beth dies, as do some 25 percent of those infected. Only in the last scene of the film is day one shown. The primary (or "index") contact is revealed to be the hapless chef, who prepared the meal of pork infected by the newly mutated virus, later shaking hands with the well-fed and unsuspecting Beth.

The rural hinterland of Hong Kong was not a coincidental choice for the origin of the new virus in *Contagion.* Each year the world prepares for a new strain of flu virus to emerge from Southeast Asia and spread through some of the largest cities on the planet, such as Hong Kong and Bangkok. The epicenter of any new epidemic is only an airplane ride away, and typically the new strains are in North America and Europe six to nine months after first appearing in Asia. Although other animal viruses are sometimes involved, mutating viruses in swine and birds are most often responsible for the thousands of recorded human flu viruses.

New human viruses must have evolved as a result of close human contact with animals ever since the dawn of primates, but until recent times they have been isolated in small localities. The onset of more frequent and rapid travel around the globe has given new viral mutations a chance to spread. It is also recognized that in the early stages of any new epidemic the case fatality rates appear to be extraordinarily high, with up to 100 percent of all infected individuals appearing to die, as only the seriously sick are brought to medical attention. Subsequent epidemic investigation invariably reveals the many additional infected persons survived or were asymptomatic, substantially reducing the case fatality rate.

In 1969, at a small mission hospital in western Nigeria, two missionary nurses became sick and rapidly died of an unexplained febrile disease. A third nurse, Lily Pinneo, also developed severe fever, came close to dying, and was transported under very trying circumstances to New York's Presbyterian Hospital. In December, a blood sample from Nurse Pinneo arrived at the Department of Epidemiology and Public Health at Yale University's School of Medicine, then the world's leading center for studying "arboviruses," those viruses spread by insects, to try and isolate the infectious agent. Professor Jordi Casals led the investigation. Three months after starting the research he developed a serious fever that could not be fully diagnosed but was thought to be Lassa fever. Casals's life was saved when he was injected with plasma containing Lassa antibodies from nurse Pinneo, then recovering in Rochester, New York. Later that year Juan Roman, a Yale laboratory technician who had not been working with the Lassa virus, went home to Pennsylvania for the Thanksgiving break where he became sick and died from a disease his doctors did not recognize but which was later confirmed to be Lassa fever. After Roman's death the viral work was transferred from Yale to the more secure biosafety labs at the CDC, precursors to the BL-4 labs prominently featured in *Contagion*.[16]

These were the first cases of Lassa fever, a disease previously unknown in the United States. The virus had mutated in Mastomys rats that live around

West African village homes and shed the virus in their urine and droppings, which when airborne could be inhaled. The same rats are also used as a food source, providing numerous opportunities for blood transmission. Widespread infection in the United States was avoided by isolating the infected patients and owing to the nature of the disease. Lassa cannot be transmitted by casual person-to-person contact but requires the exchange of body fluids, which is how the nurses were infected when caring for their patients and nursing each other. Lassa fever is now known to kill about one in five hospitalized patients but possibly as few as 1 percent of all infected individuals, many of whom remain generally asymptomatic. Since 1969, there have been several cases of visitors returning from Nigeria to the United States or Europe and shortly thereafter dying of Lassa fever. Fortunately, intensive case tracking has so far limited these infections to the index cases. Across West Africa, outbreaks of Lassa fever occur regularly, and the World Health Organization has estimated there are up to half a million infections annually in the region and some 5,000 deaths caused by the disease.

The simian immunodeficiency virus is a more widely spread infection, resulting from a mutated chimpanzee virus that does not cause disease in chimps but, as HIV, results in human AIDS. At some time in the past (it is thought between 1884 and 1914 based on molecular dating, although transmission could have occurred numerous times) this virus was passed on to African villagers, most likely from blood when preparing the chimps for food. It may have resulted in AIDS-like symptoms with high mortality, but it did not spread because the villagers were unlikely to travel far from home. Eventually, however, the disease moved beyond the African villages. It is now thought that in the 1960s a Haitian immigrant, who had worked in the Democratic Republic of the Congo where the first documented case died in 1959, brought the virus to North America.

In *Contagion* the modern methods for isolating the causative agent are represented with considerable fidelity. The infective agent is isolated from patients, and the detailed molecular structure of the virus is examined and compared to libraries of all known similar pathogens that might suggest clues as to how the disease could be treated. At the same time, vaccine developers start to model what appear to be promising vaccines. These are tested in monkeys, which have been found to be susceptible to the disease, and after much trial and error a vaccine may be found. (In *Contagion*, it was vaccine number 57.) In many actual diseases, such as Lassa fever, a vaccine has proved elusive, although for HIV, which has benefited from an extraordinary amount of research, the prospects for a vaccine are now more promising.

While emphasizing the search for a cause of the new disease, and its treatment and prevention, *Contagion* doesn't ignore the underside of life in an epidemic. A blogger (an energetic Jude Law whose blog "Truth Serum Now" is read by millions of people) promotes forsythia, a homeopathic remedy, and, worse, denounces the vaccine as being unsafe and a product of a conniving government and the pharmaceutical industry. Another shady character, a hedge fund manager looking for inside information on the future of the equity markets, appears from time to time, and there is the bureaucrat who is more interested in who will pay for the basketball court that is being appropriated to isolate patients. These situations remind us of the battles that epidemiologists must wage outside of the laboratory, the data analysis center, and the clinic when tackling a new epidemic. The constant irritants and obstacles in the search for causality will be discussed more than once in this volume.

It was difficult to demonstrate a cause of pellagra and also the causes of many of the other infectious diseases identified over the past 150 years, diseases that are now under generally successful public health control. Infections emerging from Africa and Asia will require incessant and perpetual surveillance to rapidly detect them, to understand their causes, and to find cures. Yet understanding the causes of the common chronic and complex diseases that are of most concern to people living in more technically developed countries, and finding effective and safe methods for treating them, has proven to be even more problematic. There have been frequent false dawns, many misleading leads, numerous premature breakthroughs, and therapies thought safe that later proved harmful. The perspective taken by Suzanne Shale in her description of what is expected in an Oxford University tutorial fits very nicely with how one should react to the many claims made in the scientific literature and (especially) in the press: "No beliefs are unquestionable, no statement is safe from scrutiny, no evidence is incontrovertible, and no conclusion is inescapable."[17]

The aim of this book is to demonstrate why so much published research on environmental health effects is wrong and to suggest what the reader should look for when judging whether a reported study is valid. However, a single study, with rare exceptions, should not be expected to provide sufficient evidence that an exposure causes a disease. How then should a group of studies, or indeed an entire body of literature, be reviewed to arrive at judgments about causality? This question will be examined in detail. Does the frequent occurrence of a factor, such as an environmental agent or a lifestyle behavior, with a disease infer that one is causing the other? Absolutely not! But when does an association between agent and disease become causal? This is a common dilemma in modern life and the subject of this volume. Shakespeare's Sonnet 129, the epigraph heading this chapter, is about lust and the disappointment that follows consummation. The consequences of our urge to believe in causal explanations without valid evidence, or sometimes even in spite of reliable contrary evidence, and our discomfort with uncertainty results in more than the post-coital *tristess* that Shakespeare laments. In the coming chapters we will explore the sometimes profound consequences that result from our ignoring or not understanding evidence about causation.

TWO

Chance and Randomness

Our wisdom and deliberation for the most part follow the lead of chance.
—*Michel Eyquem de Montaigne*

O! many a shaft at random sent
Find mark the archer little meant!
—*Sir Walter Scott*

Each February America celebrates its national winter pastime with an excess of testosterone-fueled activity known as the Super Bowl, when the winners of the two football conferences, National and American, compete for top dog. Interestingly, the National conference has won the Super Bowl coin toss 13 consecutive times (1998 to 2010), a result likely to happen only once in 8,192 times. Unless you believe that the NFC was able to doctor the coin, or you are convinced your dropped toast always lands with the butter side down, this has to be considered a chance result. How can that happen? If the NFC had actually won the Super Bowl 13 times in a row (they didn't, they won about half the time), that might be considered the result of good coaching, more money spent on the best players, or, depending on one's point of view, a miracle (miracles will not receive much credence in this book). Tossing a coin, however, is a random event with a probability that your call will be correct half the time. The probability of an event going forward is not the same as the probability of the totality of events looking back. Even after 12 consecutive correct calls for the coin toss, the thirteenth still had only a 50 percent chance of being correct. One is much less likely to throw 13 consecutive sixes on a die because the probability of throwing a single six is 1 out of 6 not 1 out of 2; the probability of 13 consecutive sixes is very small indeed. However, as the number of families whose children are all boys or all girls will attest, the probability of consecutive sequences of the same event, when each has a 50 percent chance of occurring, is not that uncommon.

If a string of coins landing on heads had perturbed the spectators at the games in the Greek stadia, appeals would have been made to Tyche, or in the Roman amphitheater, to Fortuna. Both were goddesses of chance and fate and wielded enormous influence in classical times. The early Greek philosophers did not believe that anything happened by chance (*automaton*) until Aristotle, who considered chance to be the simultaneous occurrence to two predetermined events. If you were accidentally struck by a flying javelin, your location had been predetermined as was the flight of the javelin. The Romans adopted the goddess Tyche, renamed her Fortuna, and her changing role in Roman life has been extensively examined. Plutarch described an ambivalent and fickle deity, who might, if so inclined, bestow good fortune on those who took risks: *Audaces fortuna iuvat* (Fortune favors the bold).[1]

Once monotheism began to dominate Western and Middle Eastern beliefs in the first centuries of the Common Era, the characteristics of the various Roman gods, not least the attributes of Fortuna, were subsumed into the one deity. The one God became the arbiter of fate, chance, and luck, and people prayed to him for protection against disease. (Given the low status of women in the desert tribes from whence these monotheistic religions arose, it is not surprising that God is always a "he.") In the Christian tradition, this near-total reliance on God to protect against illness prevailed until the Victorian period. "But deliver us from evil," the ultimate request in the Lord's Prayer, is, if nothing else, a plea for good health. With the emergence of increasingly empirical scientific knowledge, such as the understanding that filthy water and bacteria — in the water and elsewhere — were causing disease, there was a return to the more nuanced Roman view. Indeed, the Victorians thought of themselves as the new Romans: that God "helps those who help themselves." Self-improvement projects of all types were a great favorite, particularly among the Victorian elite who generally thought they didn't personally need improving but the poor did. As a result, concerns about overpopulation and food shortage led to programs that encouraged the poor to delay marriage, to have sex only to procreate, and to have smaller families.[2]

Absent other clues regarding the cause of disease, Tyche, Fortuna, and the monotheistic gods were deemed to be the agent. Of all monotheistic religions, Buddhism, which has much to commend it as a personal life style, nonetheless has, arguably, done the least to support a scientific knowledge base. Fatalism is deeply ingrained in Buddhist societies, many of which have not changed their attitudes toward disease causation since the time of the Buddha. We cannot tell if there have been improvements in the afterlife since Buddha's time, but it is certain that little has improved in their earthly lives. With modern science, the Western world has made monumental strides in understanding the causes of disease with the subsequent diminished role of chance as an explanation.

In 2009 NASA's Kepler space telescope was launched to explore the skies for extra-solar planets, with the particular goal of finding planets that may support life. These are the "Goldilocks" planets, those neither too close to their sun that they are too hot nor so far away as to be too frigid to support life. We know from our own planet how critical a distance this is, too far away and you have a polar ice cap and too close you may have the Sahara. Neither climate is completely inhospitable to life, which has moved into specialized niches in both environments, but perhaps difficult for life, at least as we know it, to have originated there. Earth is a very small planet; larger ones may have a greater range of distance from their stars and still be habitable for life, but the range remains very narrow. What is the likelihood that planets will be found where life might have evolved? There is great excitement, at the time of writing, because Kepler has newly observed some 1,200 planets with 54 probably being amenable to life. But this is a tiny fraction of what certainly exists in the universe. The telescope examined 1/400th of the sky, surveying a relatively short distance into its depths and only observing planetary orbits of four months or less; longer orbits would be missed. It is rather like standing in a forest and looking at 1 degree of the surrounding 360-degree arc only as far as the eye can see for a few hours while trying to count the number of woodpeckers in the entire woodland.

Scientists measure chance as a probability or likelihood that ranges from zero to unity (0 to 1). The extremes are rarely needed as "certainty" almost never occurs. Unless you are a neoconservative or cryo-preservationist, only taxes and death are certain; so what is the calculated probability that life will be found on another planet? It is simply a function of the number of planets. It has been estimated, with little real precision, that there are a billion billion stars across the universe. Assuming just one planet per star and that only one in a million planets is in the Goldilocks range, this indicates there are a thousand billion of them capable of supporting life. Moreover, if the chance of "intelligent life" having evolved on a Goldilocks planet is again one in a million, there are 1 million planets where this will have occurred. It takes little imagination to realize that given the age of the universe, and Homo sapiens' very short 3 million years on earth, some life forms will have had tens and perhaps hundreds of millions of years longer to evolve than ourselves. The important question is not about the existence of intelligent life elsewhere in the universe but rather where is it and has it found us yet?

What of evolution itself; is this a chance event? It seems not. With the right mix of commonplace chemicals in a Goldilocks environment, it is highly probable that strands of DNA will form resulting in an evolutionary process beginning relatively quickly. This does not mean that a tree of life will grow, like the one on earth with Homo sapiens emerging on a distant twig, but forms of life will evolve that perfectly adapt to all the ecological niches of their planet.

There are millions of alleles (single nucleotide polymorphisms [SNPs] based on four amino acids adenine, cytosine, guanine, and thymine) in the earth's life forms, and these replicate with remarkable fidelity multiple times in each cell line. But errors, called mutations, do occur either in one letter being transposed with another or in a letter or groups of letters being deleted or duplicated. How frequently this happens depends in part on the gene in which the allele resides (genes each have hundreds to thousands of alleles) and on the environment. Environmental substances, such as benzene or ionizing radiation are known to cause mutations in the genetic code; the sequence of alleles that make up the genome. These mutations are rare, and if they produce functional change in the animal or plant, then they are available for natural selection.

There is considerable randomness as to where mutations occur across the genome. Just as for the Goldilocks planets, the probability of a random event occurring is a function of both how many opportunities there are for the event to occur and how much time is given for it to occur. The 3 billion SNPs in the human genome, the hundreds of billions of cell divisions in a single lifetime, and the hundreds of millions of years it has taken for life to evolve have provided ample opportunity for evolution to occur. The resulting pattern of life that we see today in all its richness, and in the perfection of fit to its environment, may seem to be the result of a planned intelligence, what Richard Dawkins calls the Watch Maker and other people call their god. But it isn't planned. While the building blocks of evolution, the genetic mutations, are essentially random, the results they produce are subject to natural selection. This is a determined process that tests whether or not the new variation offers a selective advantage in reproduction. Evolution is an inevitable process that occurs whenever reproductive potential must meet the demands of the environment, which it always does. It is a law as certain as any law of physics, and it must be found throughout the universe wherever life, which by definition means there is reproducibility, has emerged.

Evolution is not a theory, in the sense that there is uncertainty about its main principles, any more than the theory of relativity is still a theory. It was theoretical when Charles Darwin and others introduced the concept in the mid-nineteenth century, but the early evidence from paleontology and observations in nature have been enhanced by work in physiology, molecular biology, and, most of all, genetics. Our genome is littered with evidence of an evolutionary past and in the conservation of genes that play the same roles in us as they do in fruit flies and flat worms. Perhaps the greatest argument against an intelligent designer is the "Rube Goldberg" (an American inventor of highly complex machines that perform very simple tasks) manner in which our genome has evolved from bits and pieces of genetic code put together over our evolutionary history. It is not possible to engage in modern biology or medical research without believing in evolution any more than one could be a flat earth disciple and an astronaut. Perhaps it is possible for a non-evolutionist to practice medicine, but I wonder how these doctors think antibiotic-resistant bacteria have suddenly emerged? Surely, it is easier to believe that those few mutated bacteria, newly resistant to antibiotics, were provided the opportunity to flourish in environments laden with antibiotics than it is to believe that God suddenly created them. If they weren't a problem 50 years ago, why on earth would She do that now?

Why Is the Apparent Randomness of Disease Attributed to False Causes?

Chance, randomness, and risk are all intertwined with causation. Even random events, if they have the chance to occur with sufficient frequency, may appear to have, albeit spuriously, a cause. If a large enough number of children is born with a birth defect because of a random spontaneous mutation, then enough of them will by chance have been exposed in common to some medication used by their mothers during pregnancy. If the mutation is unknown (sometimes called "silent"), the true cause of the birth defect will go unrecognized, but the medication use, which is known, may receive false attribution as the cause.

Randomness and chance can also lead to false attribution of cause when an event is rare. In the United Kingdom, a charge of murder was brought against a mother whose 2 children died from cot death (in other parts of the world called sudden infant death syndrome, or SIDS). The causes of SIDS are largely unknown although some risk factors have been identified (low birth weight, maternal smoking, and the baby sleeping on its stomach), and the occurrence appears largely random. The condition is diagnosed by exception—the child is under six months of age and no other cause of death has been identified. The probability of a child dying of SIDS is fortunately rare, about 1 in 2,000 births, but this means that there will be 350 SIDS deaths in the United Kingdom each year and the rate of having two SIDS children is 1 in 5,000,000. There are some 700,000 births annually in the United Kingdom, and so about every seven years a British mother will have

2 SIDS infants based on chance (the actual probabilities will differ based on the ratios of first to second births). In fact, the probability of SIDS recurrence in a family with SIDS in 1 child is higher than would occur simply by chance because the factors that increase risk in one pregnancy, such as maternal smoking, may continue to the next.

Sadly, these considerations were missed in cases where parents were found guilty of child murder and jailed after what must be considered statistical malpractice. The expert pediatric witness testified that the probability of a parent having multiple SIDS deaths was so small that it could not be considered a chance event. Subsequently, the Royal Statistical Society was moved to issue a clarifying statement about one particular SIDS case, and the judgment was overturned. No doubt multiple infant murders by parents do occur, but they cannot be proven based on improperly calculated probabilities that would cause the few unfortunate parents who do lose multiple babies with SIDS to be jailed by virtual lottery.

Many years ago I received a call from a Cincinnati lawyer who asked if I knew that a paper I had recently published with a colleague was being used in a legal case against a popular drug given to treat nausea in early pregnancy. This was my first introduction to Frank Woodside, a doctor turned brilliant lawyer. Frank liked to project a "country lawyer" image while engaged in highly technical and consequential legal cases, and he drew me into litigation that would eventually lead to fundamental changes in how the expert witness is viewed by the courts; this was following the US Supreme Court ruling in the Daubert case, but I am getting ahead of the story.

The paper Frank Woodside referred to examined whether the use of Bendectin (called Debendox in some countries), a demonstrably effective antinauseant drug, had increased the chance of the pregnancy resulting in a congenitally malformed child. As nausea often occurs in the early stages of pregnancy, when the fetal organs are developing, the timing was appropriate for Bendectin to be a teratogen (a substance that causes birth defects). Our paper had examined the risk on 16 various forms of malformation; 2 of them, heart valve defects and pyloric stenosis (a narrowing of the opening from the stomach to the small intestine), had suggested a positive association. How seriously should this be considered as a real finding? The signal that epidemiologists use to flag potentially important findings (usually called statistically significant and discussed in chapter 8) is, simply stated, that the chance is less than a 1 in 20 that the association observed under study is a false association. Thus, if one examines 16 congenital malformation associations, as was done in the Bendectin paper, 1 malformation is reasonably likely to meet by chance the nominal standard of statistical significance and 2 positive findings is not unexpected. In our paper, it remained uncertain whether pyloric stenosis and defective heart valves resulted from the mothers' Bendectin use.[3]

Of course, it was remotely possible that Bendectin might cause these particular (unrelated) malformations and not others. Some drugs do cause specific types of malformation; for example, sodium valproate, a common antiepileptic drug, causes the malformation spina bifida. The epidemiologist's dilemma is how to determine which explanation for the observed association is most likely correct. The first step (we consider the determination of causation in detail in chapter 15) is to rule out chance as an explanation for the association.[4] Sorting out true associations from those occurring by chance is much more than a statistical exercise; a key consideration is whether the observed association is replicated in other studies. For pyloric stenosis or heart valve defects and Bendectin, there was no consistent replication by other investigators, and so our finding of an association must be considered to have occurred by chance.

Bendectin was used, worldwide over many years, by some 30 million pregnant women. Given the normal congenital malformation rate occurring in 3–5 percent of pregnancies, chance alone determined that some 1 million women who had used Bendectin would go on to deliver a baby with a congenital anomaly. Bendectin-exposed, congenitally malformed children, with every type of organ anomaly, were not uncommon and provided many litigants for a class action lawsuit. We will pick up more details of the Bendectin case when we explore issues of causality and harm. The unhappy ending of this story is that while the manufacturers of Bendectin won the class action suit of 1,300 plaintiffs defended by Frank Woodside, and almost every other lawsuit, the cost of litigation and increased insurance premiums forced the manufacturer to stop production of the drug. At the present time, to treat women's nausea in pregnancy, doctors use other medications about which much less is known as to their safety or effectiveness. In the spring of 2011, 25 years after the vexatious Bendectin litigation, it was reported that in Britain nausea and vomiting in pregnancy was being "trivialized" by doctors who were afraid to prescribe drugs to treat it because there is still no formally licensed drug and doctors were afraid of being blamed for any birth defects.[5]

On another occasion, while at a scientific meeting, I saw a report purportedly linking spermicide contraception exposure and congenital malformations. This report, however, was not presented at a scientific session; instead it appeared on *Good Morning America*, a popular television morning talk show. In what must be a prime example of editorial misjudgment, *JAMA*, a highly respected medical journal, had published an account of four children, each born with a (different) congenital malformation after possibly being exposed to their mother's use of spermicides. Spermicides are one of the most widely used forms of contraception, and because they are frequently ineffective, millions of women deliver potentially exposed babies. Given the extensive use of spermicides, it is not unusual to have babies with malformations born after exposure to them. Bendectin and spermicides both illustrate where the search for causality can lead to misleading results. (I will discuss other examples of misleading studies in the pages ahead.)

One, perhaps predictable, consequence of publishing the spermicide paper in a leading medical journal, whose contributions are widely publicized, became clear when I returned to my university and learned that the hospital had seen a spike in women requesting induced abortions. As a result of the press coverage from this paper, and knowing they had conceived while using spermicides and fearing a malformed child, some women elected to abort an otherwise wanted conception. Sadly, ultrasonography and other currently used tests were not then widely available to provide these mothers with more accurate information about the health of their fetus.

When there are multiple opportunities for a chance event to happen, the event will eventually occur. This is why many see images of the Virgin Mary in the clouds or on tree bark: countless clouds and trees are observed by millions of people and images of all kinds are perceived. Every Saturday, thousands of coins are tossed to determine which sports team will kick off first, creating an untold number of opportunities for consecutive coin toss wins by one team.

There are tens of thousands of doctors seeing millions of patients every day and it should come as no surprised that some of them will see several patients with the same medical condition who have been exposed to the same environmental agent or lifestyle choice. Clinicians often publish these observations as "letters to the editor," and the medical journal the *Lancet* is one of the most popular places to find them. The letters are not considered by the health professions to be evidence that the cause of a disease has been identified; there have been too many false alarms for that and the fallibility of case reports is well understood. However, they create hypotheses for further study, and some, a small but important minority of case reports, do turn out to be supported by more rigorous research. Letters suggesting that women who used oral contraceptives, especially in conjunction with smoking, were at greater risk for stroke were proven to be correct; however, other letters reporting an increased risk of congenital malformations after oral contraceptive use were not subsequently supported.

Anne Anderson, the mother of a child being treated for leukemia at a Boston hospital, was surprised to meet several other mothers of children being similarly treated from the same Massachusetts town, Woburn, where she lived. Encouraged, quite appropriately, by this observant mother, a series of extensive but ultimately inconclusive studies to try and identify a common source of exposure to these children was undertaken. Analysis of several years' cancer statistics showed higher rates of leukemia, with 20 cases in the cluster area. The primary culprits were solvents, arsenic, and heavy metal contamination of the water supply in two of several wells (wells G and H) supplying water to the area of Woburn with the leukemia cluster. These contaminants were likely the product of a large nineteenth-century tanning industry in Woburn that made leather belts and shoes for Civil War soldiers. The Woburn leukemia cluster led to a best-selling book and movie,[6] adding to a heated and inflammatory environment, the kind that can hinder the investigation of disease clusters.

A detailed study of the Woburn water supply by Harvard biostatisticians showed that homes with affected children were twice as likely to have had some water supplied by wells G and H than were homes of children outside the cluster. By the time their analysis was completed, wells G and H had been closed down, and another analysis showed that the leukemia rates had subsequently returned to normal in the cluster area. Was this sufficient evidence to show the cluster had not occurred by chance? Like every other major leukemia cluster that has been studied by the Centers for Disease Control, a direct link with the water contaminants, some of which are a known cause of leukemia, was never conclusively demonstrated. The cause of the cluster was never satisfactorily explained, and like most clusters, it declined over time. Childhood leukemia is a rare disease, affecting 1 to 2 children for every 10,000 in the United States, but it rarely spreads evenly across a community. Rather it appears to "cluster" in unpredictable ways that may suggest some underlying pattern reflecting causation. Unfortunately, for the investigating epidemiologist, these patterns almost always cluster by chance, not because of any underlying common environmental exposure.[7]

In my own small town on the Connecticut shore, a cancer cluster was claimed to have occurred on Meadow Street. It was no coincidence that Meadow Street had a small electrical generator and this claim was made at a time when there was growing concern that non-ionizing electromagnetic fields (EMF) could cause cancer. California schools had been closed and homes could not be sold because of their close proximity to power lines. The *New Yorker* magazine published a lengthy series of articles by Paul Brodeur, known previously for writing extensively about the never proven, but he claimed dangerous, health effects of radar. The residents of Meadow Street identified four homes that had a history of four different kinds of cancer and attributed this to EMF from the power plant. In fact, a careful survey of any street in the town would likely produce the same proportion of families with a cancer history. This was an imaginary cluster planted in the minds of innocent people by a fevered journalist who should have known better.

In the United States tornadoes are more common in Oklahoma and surrounding areas (in what is called "tornado alley") than they are in New England. But within Oklahoma, the chance of being struck by a tornado is random, regardless of where one lives in the state. This is a spatial aspect of chance. Similarly, because of changes in annual weather patterns, one year may see more tornadoes than others. In some years the chance of being struck by a tornado, while still random, is greater than in other years. This is a temporal component. We will see that studying disease clusters poses challenges due to the difficulty in sampling both time and space (chapter 9). If the size of the cluster is expanded to a larger area, and pushed back or forward in time, the increased rate of disease will usually disappear. This could reflect changes in exposure and be of genuine interest, but it most likely demonstrates the chance nature of the cluster. The smaller the area that is examined, or the briefer the time period studied, the less opportunity there is for randomness to become apparent. If lightning strikes someone under a tree, and we study only that one tree, it appears as if that particular tree has characteristics that encouraged the strike. Perhaps it is taller, has a thicker trunk, or is situated on a hill, all of which may be falsely attributed to encouraging the strike. If we study all the neighboring trees we may find others that were not struck despite having the same attributes, making us more willing to accept the chance nature of the strike.

Similarly, it may be thought that a cancer cluster among a group of workers is caused by the chemicals to which they are exposed, and indeed it might be. But before a causal attribution can be made, it is necessary to look at workers in other places who are exposed to the same chemicals and to also extend the observation period back in time to see if the higher disease rates occurred earlier (and perhaps to follow the cluster forward in time to see if the higher disease rates persist). If the higher disease rates are observed in other similar work places and they persist over time, then a "true" cluster may have been identified. If it does not, the initial cluster was almost certainly a chance event.

Chance events are translated into "real" associations in our minds when the timing of an illness seems closely connected to a prior event. A mother whose child's vaccination is followed within a couple of days by a seizure or some other unanticipated neurological condition, one which perhaps leads to a diagnosis of autism, must be forgiven for connecting the one with the other. The rarity of the neurological condition further adds to her certainty that it was caused by the vaccination. Although they merit investigation, these two events are most likely just co-incident in time; they are literally coincidental.

Box 2.1. Margaux Bubble Security Tags.

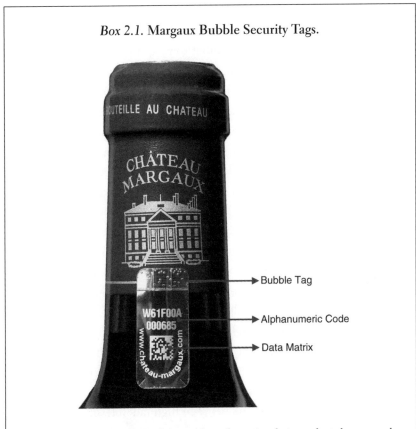

The Margaux Vineyards, and those of us who enjoy their product, have a problem with forgeries of their label being used by others and placed on bottles of cheaper wine. To make forgeries more difficult, Margaux developed a bubble security tag that uniquely labels each bottle and allows the vineyard to track individual bottles. The label is the product of the random formation of bubbles; no two are the same but all of them show clusters of bubbles within the pattern. Indeed, it is the clustering that makes each label unique. If we overlay two authentic Margaux labels, there will be areas where the bubble clusters overlap.

We know that both environmental exposures and disease prevalence occur in clusters, and given a large enough area, some clusters of exposure and of disease will overlap. Without knowing the complete pattern of these clusters, the overlapping but random clusters will appear as a strong association between exposure and disease rather than the chance associations they most likely are.

Photograph Courtesy of Margaux Vineyards.

Again the broader probabilities need to be understood: there are millions of children vaccinated annually and thousands of them have seizures or develop autism. It is to be expected that some of these events will collide; many seizures will occur by chance and within a few days or even hours following the vaccination. There has been enormous public concern as to whether childhood vaccination leads to a variety of health outcomes. The scientific evidence *against* any association between them is very strong, but the individual cases seem very suggestive to those involved. Unfortunately, this concern has resulted in mothers not vaccinating their children and in subsequent epidemics of measles, a disease that can have serious and life-threatening consequences for children. The same misattributions are seen when sudden infant (or crib) death occurs after vaccination or when strokes and myocardial infarctions follow flu shots in the elderly. Only detailed study of tens of thousands of records reveals that these events are really not linked together and are just the result of chance association.

If we examine enough schools, some will show higher levels of radon than others; some will have higher rates of leukemia than others, and a few will experience high rates of both. (Some will also have lower levels of radon and less leukemia than expected, but these are never brought to the public's attention.) Only by looking at sufficiently large numbers of schools can we ascertain whether the link between high radon levels and increased leukemia risk is replicated in more schools than would be expected by chance and whether the observed "risky" school was so categorized following a random event.

At any one time around the world, millions of women are using some form of oral contraception and also attending thousands of medical practices. Some of these practices will see an unusually large number of their patients who are using a particular type of oral contraceptive. Let's make up a name and call it Ovule. Some other medical practices will see an unusually large number of patients who have developed early onset breast cancer, and given the large number of medical practices, some will see an excess of Ovule users who also develop breast cancer. Are these random events, or is there an association between Ovule and early onset breast cancer? If enough doctors write up their observation and send it to a medical journal,

Box 2.2 Some Things That Appear Random Are Not.

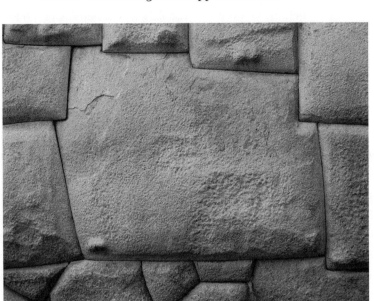

Some events that appear to be random are actually deterministic. The famous 12-sided Inca block in Cuzco, Peru, looks like a random configuration, but it is, in fact, carefully constructed to take into account the existing blocks in the wall and others that will be placed on top of it. This stone is also a "male stone" because it has prominences that attach it to the adjacent "female" stones. The ability of this style of construction to avoid earthquake damage is legendary. In a quake, the stones move over each other but do not collapse. In contrast, the Catholic temples built on top of the Inca foundations but using European methods fell several times over the centuries. Another example of an apparently random pattern is illustrated in the vein structures of a leaf, which are actually determined by their function and have evolved to maximize the efficient delivery of nutrients to the entire surface of the leaf.

Photograph by Maryann Bracken.

they will encourage the start of systematic study. Only by conducting a study in thousands, or possibly tens of thousands, of women will it be possible to determine whether the observed association between Ovule and breast cancer was a random event or if there seems to be a real association. Even if the association is real, whether Ovule actually *causes* breast cancer and how that is investigated is the topic of future chapters.

Why Do Diseases with Determined Cause Appear Random?

Why do some diseases appear to be random and due to chance when they actually have a determined cause? Any disease whose cause is unknown will appear to be occurring by chance, and all new disease epidemics exemplify this. Only after the natural history of the disease is understood will a causal agent be shown to account for what had seemed to be the apparently random occurrences. Around 1900, typhoid was one of the great killers in New York City, especially among the squalor of the Lower East Side tenements filled with immigrants from Europe. Among the poor, the disease appeared to strike by chance. Only when the role of typhoid carriers was understood (people who did not have symptoms but who carried and passed on the disease, the most infamous being a cook, "typhoid Mary" Mallon), did it become clearer why some people but not others were infected with the disease.[8]

The same phenomenon occurred in the 1854 London cholera epidemic. Before John Snow demonstrated that water from one particular pump on Broad Street was contaminated, the patterns of disease in the immediate area around the pump had a random character. Snow carefully mapped the cholera cases in a larger area of London and made several insightful observations. For example, there was an absence of cholera among local brewery workers who had easy access to an alternative beverage; and the occurrence of cholera in a lady who lived some distance away from Broad Street but drank water from the pump, preferring the taste, while no other cases occurred in her neighborhood. Snow showed a pattern of disease that was far from random and not due to chance. He fully deserves his reputation as the first modern observational epidemiologist.

In the early stages of the AIDS epidemic in 1981, when symptoms first started to appear in the San Francisco male gay community, investigating epidemiologists saw what appeared to be an increasing but random pattern of two normally rare diseases (Kaposi's sarcoma and Pneumocystis carinii pneumonia or Pneumocystis jiroveci pneumonia). For two years, until the discovery of the HIV virus in France, the real cause of the disease was unknown. It was not for another year and after the virus was also identified in the United States that the disease was confirmed as being sexually transmitted and its occurrence began to form a more coherent pattern.[9]

There are still many diseases that today appear to us to occur by chance. There are rare mutations that produce conditions such as tetralogy of Fallot (which has four developmental errors in the heart) and other serious heart malformations. Why do these occur in a small minority of people (about 1 in 3,000) but not in others? These occurrences appear to be random because we do not know why the spontaneous mutations occur (they do not appear in families). In a flu epidemic, we do not fully understand why some people show none of the flu symptoms even though they were exposed to the flu virus. With our lack of understanding, the disease appears to affect people by chance. Discovering the real cause of disease, so that randomness disappears and patterns of real causation emerge, is the science of epidemiology. But as we will see throughout this book, many missteps can occur on the way to that more complete understanding.

Why are we so eager to adopt associations as being causal even when there is no evidence to support that conclusion? Why are we unwilling to accept uncertainty until such a time as evidence has been developed that can provide a firm conclusion? Has our evolution favored a less cautious and questioning approach? Michael Shermer, the founding publisher of *Skeptic* magazine, has postulated that assumptions of causality, even if premature, have survival value. Apes and early hominoids who thought the rustling grass was simply due to the wind were much more likely to die and not pass on their "incautious" genes than the individual who worried that the grass was disturbed by a lion and fled up a tree.

Of course, climbing a tree every time the grass rustled would produce a very tired and hungry hominoid who might also have difficulty passing on his genes. This would offer only a slight advantage of one behavior over the other but still sufficient, many generations later, to result in a species predestined to jump to a conclusion about causes. Indeed, it has been suggested that our propensity to deny chance as the explanation for events, when not knowing the real cause, may explain the seemingly ubiquitous need for humans to create deities to explain that which otherwise remains inexplicable. As Sébastien Chamfort put it: "Chance is a nickname for Providence." And Anatole France: "Chance is perhaps the pseudonym of God when he did not want to sign." In short, God did not create us in his image but rather we created God in ours.

When the great New England hurricane of 1938 suddenly appeared on September 21 as a category 3 storm, early warnings having been ignored, it appeared to many onlookers to be "fate," a "chance" occurrence, or as the insurance adjusters still would have it, "an act of God." In contrast, when Hurricane Irene arrived on August 28, 2011, it was a much-anticipated event. First tracked by satellite as a tropical wave emerging from the Sahara Desert, then building to a tropical depression before becoming a hurricane at landfall, Irene was followed for several weeks and landfall accurately predicted within hours and a few miles. Familiarity with "steering currents," central wall collapse, precise tracking, and accurate wind speed calculations all contributed to a greater understanding of the storm. Consequently, preparations could be made, evacuations completed, and major loss of life avoided. This seemed much less of a chance event and more a natural and explicable phenomenon.

Chance is widely considered to be a real phenomenon; whether a thrown die turns up a six or any other number between one and five is a chance event, provided no one has fiddled with the die. However, chance is also the explanation given to events that reflect our lack of knowledge about what causes them. Scientists call this "random error" and try to account for it in their explanatory models that attempt to predict the likelihood of an event, like a disease, occurring. Kenneth Rothman has described this as being "part of our experience that we cannot predict."[10] A less gentle way of putting it is that chance reflects our ignorance of the true causes of an event. It may be that there will always be a chance element in our understanding of causation, we cannot claim that we will ever know everything about everything or even about anything, but the role of chance will diminish as our understanding grows. The goal of science in seeking causal explanations is to reduce the role of chance to as small a component of the causal pathways as possible. As the role of chance is reduced, prediction becomes more precise.

It is no accident that the dominance of religion and superstition (some would not make a distinction) in explaining natural events, including the occurrence of disease, has diminished as the scientific paradigm has evolved over the last four hundred years. Some surveys estimate over 90 percent of professional biologists claim to be atheists whereas only 10 percent of the general population do so. Indeed, Richard Dawkins, one of the most controversial biologists of our time famously commented that: "We are all atheists about most of the gods that humanity has ever believed in. Some of us just go one god further."[11] The reasons for this would seem obvious: biologists understand in a very profound way how patterns of life have evolved to perfectly fit their "ecological niche," why an osprey or salmon always returns to the same nesting site after a 2,000-mile migration. Biologists see little need to resort to explanations of fate, or chance, or acts of God.

Randomness reflects our failure to understand all the causal influences on a phenomenon. We know that throwing six dice will produce an apparently random variation of 462 possible combinations of numbers, and we are content not to have to understand what might "cause" certain patterns to occur more frequently than others, that is, to influence the randomness (how the dice are placed in the shaker, how they are shaken, what angle they hit the gaming table, and so on). However, in trying to understand natural phenomena that are important to us, such as why someone develops cancer and someone else does not, we do seek to understand and reduce the apparently random occurrences of disease, and the more we understand them the less we believe disease is a random or chance occurrence.

Our continuing lack of a full understanding of disease etiology, and yet a belief that there must be some cause for all the ill health that afflicts us even though what that is remains not fully understood, has resulted in numerous premature and spurious claims of causality. Environmental agents or some aspect of our life styles causes this or that illness. These claims are motivated by our unwillingness to accept uncertainty. While chance and randomness still plague much of the science of epidemiology, we will see in a later chapter how randomness has been harnessed to create one of the most important powerful scientific breakthroughs in history: the development of the randomized controlled trial.

THREE

Risk

Men's most valuable trait is a judicious sense of what not to believe.
—*Euripides, 480–406* BCE

The first two days of our cruise saw little wind and an uneventful pas-
sage east from our home port in Casco Bay, first to Christmas Cove
in South Bristol a favored sailors' watering hole with a bar full of ancient
burgees from yacht clubs worldwide, and the next day across Muscongus
Bay to Allen Island, home of the Wyeth painters, and into Penobscot Bay.
Only as we sailed north up Muscle Ridge Channel in the early afternoon
did we see a fog bank rolling in from the south, not an unusual occurrence
and not of concern as Dix Island was off to starboard. That familiar bay a
few minutes away beckoned, and a quiet afternoon at anchor seemed preferable to closely monitoring the chart plotter through a rocky channel. No
sooner was the anchor set than visibility dropped to a few yards and the
wind died. Suddenly, torrential rain and heavy lightning were upon us, and
an hour later the storm really hit, now with increasing wind and forked
lightning strikes all around and a continuous play of sheet lightning that
illuminated impressive white caps in the anchorage. This was clearly no
ordinary storm.

By evening the rain continued unabated and the wind whined through
the rigging as *Nordic Spirit* tugged violently at her anchor, pitching and rolling wildly. The anchorage was fully exposed to the north where the wind,
most unusually for this time of year, was coming from. When we had an-
chored at mid-tide, 60 feet of rode in 20 feet of water seemed adequate, but
now it was high tide and more line would have to be let out. Darkness had

fallen early and with so much spray it was impossible to tell water from the air. I put on the spreader lights to illuminate the deck, decided against a harness which could have hung me up on the deck fittings, opened the hatch, and was immediately soaked with rain and flying spray. To avoid being pitched overboard, I crawled on hands and knees to the bow. The anchor rode was tight as a bowstring. Untying the anchor line, it immediately ran out a hundred feet before I could get a turn back around the cleat. Another 40 feet was let out and the boat's pitching immediately seemed less extreme. I crawled back to the cockpit, with lightning still dancing all around and the wind intensifying to a wildness I had never seen before.

Back in the cabin we watched the boat's position on the GPS chart plotter. She seemed to be holding position although swinging in an alarmingly wide arc. Several minutes later, the wind, spray, and lightning intensified in one final angry burst before subsiding with surprising rapidity to a light breeze. We had held.[1]

That evening off the Maine coast didn't lend itself to serious etymological discussion. I subsequently settled down with a scotch and only much later appreciated that we had experienced what may have been the source of the concept of risk. The ancient Greeks are thought to have used the navigational term *rhīza*, perhaps metaphorically, for sailing dangerously close to the rocks, or cliffs, and the Latin *resegāreis* derived from coastal rocks appearing shear out of the water. Odysseus lost his ship on the cliffs of Scylla in a storm brought on by Zeus.[2]

Humans have evolved with risk, it is an integral component of natural selection: the chirp of the chick can alert its mother to feed it but also the hovering hawk to feed on it. Lionesses give birth a distance away from the pride but must decide when to introduce their cubs to the other members of the pride: if the male lions accept them, they are protected, but if not they will be killed. The lioness has no choice but to accept the risk to her cubs. Mothers throughout history must have taken the risk of feeding themselves and leaving their newborns unattended. Risk is ubiquitous and it is relative. The risk of one course of action is always: compared to what? Risk is popularly thought to be an absolute: say, what is the risk of rock climbing? But we must consider what this is being compared to: the risk of staying in bed, trekking, or hang gliding? The Greek sailor, and every navigator since, had to risk sailing next to the rocky shore with relatively calmer waters versus the rougher offshore waters and fewer obstacles. So, what is risk relative to?

Risk as a Relative Construct

Risk, and how it is expressed, is far from a simple concept. It can be relative to some other exposure or course of action, it can be an observed risk compared to an expected or standard risk, or it may be calculated as a lifetime risk or risk per year. Determining causality requires an assessment of relative risk. If an environmental factor is to be examined for the strength of its association with a disease, the risk of disease after exposure must be compared to the risk without exposure. Similarly, in the evaluation of a therapeutic drug to see if it "causes" recovery from illness, there must be a comparison to recovery without the drug or with using another one. Not surprising, then, *relative* risk is the most important measure of risk used by epidemiologists and health professionals in their studies of causality. (The calculation is straightforward: if there is a 1 percent chance of dying over the next year based on population data but among people who drink a bottle of whisky a day the chance is 5 percent, the relative risk of death from very heavy whisky drinking is 5 ($RR = 5$, 5 divided by 1).) Despite its importance, the concept of relative risk did not enter the scientific vocabulary until relatively recently.[3]

The pellagra research papers discussed earlier are free of any calculations of relative risk; the raw numbers were expected to tell the story. Indeed all through the 1940s and 1950s there was almost no mention of relative risk in scientific research. Occasionally the prevalence rate of disease in one group would be compared with the prevalence rate in another with the comment that one rate was so many times larger than that of the other, which is a measure of relative risk, but it was not so identified. The first detailed description of relative risk and its preference as the measure of risk in making determinations about causality is attributed to Jerome Cornfield, a prominent biostatistician at the National Cancer Institute in Washington who was writing at the same time that the causal relationship of cigarette smoking with lung cancer was being debated. Despite publication in 1950 of the (now considered classic) studies of Richard Doll and Bradford Hill in the United Kingdom, and Ernst Wynder and Evarts Graham in the United States, there were prominent voices, chief among them R. A. Fisher (perhaps the leading biostatistician of his generation), suggesting that the association of smoking with lung cancer was not real but was likely confounded by other behavioral, life style, and especially genetic factors.[4]

Cornfield and his colleagues demonstrated that for any other (confounding) factor to be able to explain the risk of smoking, the ratio of the prevalence of a confounding factor in the smokers relative to the prevalence of that factor in the nonsmokers must exceed the relative risk for the suspected causal agent.[5] The relative risk for smoking and lung cancer was approximately 15, and so the prevalence of any confounding factor would need to occur more than 15 times in smokers compared to nonsmokers. In fact, such a confounding factor should be easy to detect in a well-designed epidemiological study and is unlikely to remain unobserved for long, even if not initially studied. Fisher believed that the hidden confounder, which he was never able to identify, was probably of genetic origin. We now know that such large relative risks are uncommon in genetic associations (discussed in chapter 10), but Fisher's view failed to gain widespread support for other considerations. A contentious argument in Cornfield's time was whether or not smoking was a cause of cardiovascular deaths. Whereas smoking increased lung cancer risk by 15 to 30 times, for cardiovascular disease it was only doubled. The size of the relative risk is influenced by the prevalence of the disease in the unexposed population; it is quite possible to achieve a high relative risk when the baseline risk is 1/1,000 but mathematically impossible if the baseline risk is, say, 300/1,000 (in this latter case the highest possible relative risk is 3.3).

Cornfield and colleagues did not see a role for using absolute risk in assessing causality; to them "the absolute measure would be important in appraising the public health significance of an effect known to be causal." To this day, this is the most commonly described utility of the relative and absolute measures of risk. Recently Charles Poole, an influential theoretical epidemiologist, provided the proof missed by Cornfield: that risk difference

can be interpreted in the same way as relative risk. If a confounder is to explain a proposed causal association, the *difference* between the prevalence
of the confounder in the exposed versus unexposed groups must be greater
than the risk difference between the causal agent and the unexposed. This
is especially useful where the prevalence of disease is quite high and the
risk differences are correspondingly smaller. Poole has argued that failure to
recognize the importance of the risk difference was responsible for the delayed recognition, now widely accepted, that smoking was causally related
to cardiovascular disease.[6]

Sodium valproate, a drug prescribed to treat epilepsy, has been used for
many years and is known to be very effective in controlling epileptic seizures.
When women who suffer from epilepsy become pregnant, it is particularly
important that their seizures are controlled as seizure activity during pregnancy can endanger the survival of the fetus. It is generally considered that
using valproate in early pregnancy, compared to using another antiepileptic
drug, increases the risk of the child being born with incomplete closure of
the spinal column, a condition known as spina bifida. This congenital malformation requires surgery and carries not inconsiderable risk of permanent
disability to the child. How can the risk of this condition be described to
epileptic mothers using valproate?

It is well established that the normal occurrence of spina bifida is about
1.5 times in every 1,000 births.[7] Several studies have shown that the risk
to children of women using valproate compared to the children of those
not using any antiepileptic drug rises to at least 15 per 1,000 births. The
increased risk, which as we have seen is called the relative risk because the
risk in babies exposed to valproate is assessed relative to those unexposed,
is about 10. How is the relative risk interpreted to help patients and doctors
decide whether or not to use valproate during pregnancy? The additional
risk of spina bifida over the background rate, incurred by using valproate,
is 13.5/1,000; this is also called the risk difference ($15 - 1.5 = 13.5$). The risk
of having a child with spina bifida after exposure to valproate is some 13.5
per thousand beyond the baseline risk (the probability is 0.0135). Dividing
13.5 into 1,000 gives 74 which is called the number needed to harm (NNH).
This tells us that of every 74 pregnant women treated with valproate, one

might be expected to have a child with spina bifida that is caused by the drug. NNH is a readily understood statistic, often used by policy makers as well as clinicians to make decisions about the use of medical drugs.

We cannot underestimate the importance of considering the size of the relative risk in making conclusions about causality. The small farming community of Cândido Godói in Brazil has a rate of twins some 10 times the normal rate of twin births (normally about 1 twin birth per 80 singleton births, although the twinning rate is higher in recent times, probably due to artificial reproductive technologies used to enhance the chance of conception). The Cândido Godói twinning rate, with a relative risk of 10, is much higher than reportedly elevated twinning rates in other parts of the world. It provides strong evidence that some particular risk factor is raising the rate and that this is not simply due to chance. Interestingly, in Cândido Godói there had been a suspicion that the twinning rate was the result of the town once being the home of Josef Mengele, who practiced medicine as Rudolf Weiss following his escape from Nazi Germany where he had conducted horrific medical experiments on the inmates of concentration camps. Mengele had a particular fascination with twins and saw them as a way to increase the rate of Aryan birth for the Third Reich. Since the twins in Candido Godoi were typically blond haired and had light-colored eyes, speculation was rife that Mengele was somehow responsible. The real cause of the increased twinning was recently reported by Ursula Matte, a Brazilian geneticist who studied records from the area that showed the high twinning rates predated Mengele living there, but she also identified a genetic variant in the population. The impact of the variant was enhanced because of a high level of inbreeding in the immigrant population, many of whom were of German origin. This presumably accounts for the high rate of "Aryan" twins and perhaps why Mengele settled there in the first place.[8]

Some relative risks are so large that there can be no doubt they reflect a causal association. Following are two examples.

The human reproductive system has evolved so that of the several hundred thousand sperm ejaculated at intercourse, only one is used for conception of a single egg. After the first sperm has entered the ovum, the surrounding membrane immediately changes its structure to prevent additional sperms from passing through. Like all biological systems, this is not perfect and occasionally two sperms enter the ovum (called dispermy), which results in a molar (also called hydatidiform mole) pregnancy. Most molar pregnancies, called partial moles, have a chromosomal make up that is XXY (compared with XX and XY in the normal female and male, respectively). A second type of molar pregnancy, called a complete molar pregnancy, may also result from dispermy but mostly derives from the fertilization of an ovum where the female genetic material is lost and both of the X chromosomes come from the father. Women who experience a complete molar pregnancy are 1,000 to 2,000 times more likely to develop a serious and sometimes fatal cancer called choriocarcinoma, a tumor of the tissue that forms the placenta. Instead of a usual risk of 1 in 40,000 pregnancies being followed by choriocarcinoma, after a complete molar pregnancy the risk is 1 in 40 pregnancies or higher. The evidence that complete molar pregnancies cause most choriocarcinoma is enhanced by a lack of other strong associations with the disease. Except for extremes in maternal age, no other risk factors for choriocarcinoma have been identified.[9]

In the late 1950s and early 1960s a large number of babies were born with severely deformed, shortened, or missing limbs, a condition known as phocomelia (after the Greek word for "seal limbs"). This condition is extremely rare and the sudden increase in its prevalence suggested a new prenatal exposure was most likely responsible. Investigations indicated that a new pregnancy drug, prescribed as a sedative and used for morning sickness, might be the culprit. The drug was thalidomide. Most phocomelia malformations, up to 2,500 of them, occurred in Germany where thalidomide, under the brand name Contergan, had been actively promoted by the Chemie Grünenthal Company. The baseline rate of the condition is around 1 per million births and results from a rare genetic condition. Indeed, it is extremely unusual to find cases of phocomelia that were not exposed to thalidomide. After exposure to thalidomide, the risk was estimated to be between 20 percent and 40 percent that suggests a relative risk of at least 200,000 indicating an unequivocal causal relationship.[10]

Risk may of course be decreased rather than increased with exposure to some risk factors. Thousands of published studies examine the use of nutritional supplements to see if they reduce the risk of various diseases but especially cancer. The goal of many clinical trials is also to determine whether or not the treatment of interest lowers the severity of disease or decreases mortality. How should we view the size of a "protective" relative risk? It will be immediately obvious that the spread of relative risk around one (called "unity" or no risk) is not symmetrical. Relative risks greater than unity can range from one to infinity; we have discussed some relative risks in the hundreds and thousands. A relative risk of 2 is a 100 percent increase in risk, 10 is a 900 percent increased risk, and relative risk of 100 is 9900 percent increased risk. In contrast, a relative risk less than unity can range only from one to zero. Protective effects can be no greater than 100 percent.[11]

I have argued that relative risks greater than 10 are powerful evidence that the exposure of interest may actually have some causal role in the disease under study. This assumes, of course that some reasonable precautions against study bias were taken (which are described in chapter 6) and that other studies have found a similar result. There are no equivalent thresholds for protective effects. If a nutritional supplement were shown, in an observational study, to reduce the risk of disease by 80 percent (RR=0.20) that would be considered a very strong effect. If the same result were observed in a large randomized trial, which as we will see is much freer of bias, this would be considered a remarkable result. But smaller "protective effects" seen in observational studies, as discussed later, are readily the result of bias and cannot on their face value provide any assessment of causality without additional careful study and replication. In contrast, for some randomized trials a reduction in risk of only 10 percent or less may be considered to be important, particularly if the exposure is widespread. This is further discussed in chapter 5.

For some diseases it is helpful to calculate lifetime risk; that is, over the course of a typical life what is the risk of the disease occurring. The average lifetime risk of breast cancer for women in the United States is about 12 percent. Other risks may be calculated as an annual rate, for example, what is the average *annual* risk of developing cancer? For breast cancer it is between 1 and 2 per thousand women. In one of his superb weekly columns on "Bad Science" in the *Guardian* newspaper, Ben Goldacre showed how risk estimates can be very misleading if the correct denominator is not applied.[12] In his example, the British press had widely reported 584 pregnancies occurring in women who were using a contraceptive implant, suggesting poor effectiveness. However, the implants had been used for over ten years and the United Kingdom Medicines and Health Care Products Regulatory Agency estimated that 1.4 million implants had been sold. Since each implant was used for about three years, the total exposure time was actually 4.1 million woman-years at risk. Goldacre described the correct way in which epidemiologists calculate this type of risk (based on person-years of exposure) and points out that the actual failure rate of the contraceptive implant is 1.4 per 10,000 woman-years at risk, indicating it is actually one of the most effective methods of contraception.

Risk permeates all aspects of medicine. There is a risk from all medical therapies that they will harm rather than cure. Every medicine produces negative reactions in some people. An old adage, attributed to Paracelsus, has it that "Poison is in everything, and no thing is without poison. The dosage makes it either a poison or a remedy." At high enough doses every medicine is toxic, but it is more complicated than that. Even at therapeutic levels, all medicines are harmful to a select group of people: this may depend on a person's genetic makeup and also on the foods they eat (people

---

Box 3.1. Integrating Therapeutic Benefit with Risk.

Consider a therapy for stroke that reduces the baseline risk from 4.3 percent to 0.9 percent. The risk difference is 3.4 percent and the number needed to treat (NNT) is $100/3.4 = 29$.

If the number of important bleeds incurred by the therapy is 1 percent, we can calculate the risk benefit from the therapy as $29 \times 0.01 = 0.29$. That is, the therapy results in one important bleed for every three prevented strokes.*

In a real clinical situation the risk of several complications may need to be estimated for a complete quantification of the benefits and risks.

*Data calculated from Ezekowitz MD, James KE. Stroke prevention in atrial fibrillation II study. Lancet. 1994;343(8911):1508–1509.

---

on anticholesterol medicines must avoid grapefruit), other medicines they take (oral contraceptives interfere with several drugs, including antidepressants and beta-blockers), or whether they smoke. The interactions of many drugs with diet are well known. One of the goals of modern pharmacological research is to identify patients who will benefit from a drug and not suffer harmful side effects.

What Is Acceptable Risk?

There is much debate as to how much risk from an effective therapy should be tolerated, and the degree of acceptable risk depends on several factors. Rosiglitazone is a drug developed to bring blood sugar under stricter control in diabetic patients, and given good evidence that it is successful in lowering levels of glycemia, it became one of the most commonly prescribed of all drugs. Several years after it had been approved by regulatory agencies, some researchers observed that the drug increased the risk of myocardial infarction by about 30 percent and death by about 15 percent compared to patients receiving another type of "glitazone" drug. These increased risks were seen in analyses of all the evidence from randomized trials and in systematic reviews of all observational studies. There seems little doubt that the risks are causal and the increase in death is estimated at about 43 excess deaths for every 10,000 patients using Rosiglitazone. This is an unacceptable risk for three major reasons: diabetes is common (between 8 and 9 percent of the US population has diabetes) and a large number of people will be exposed to risk; tighter glycemic control does not appear to bring additional health benefits, and another drug of similar effectiveness is available with a safer risk profile.[13]

One factor influencing how much risk is acceptable is whether the condition can be managed using an alternative medication. If a cholesterol-reducing or blood pressure–lowering drug is causing a problem in some patients, there are several other drugs available and so tolerance for any complications is low. In contrast, there are few therapeutic options for treating HIV/AIDS and so higher complication rates are tolerated. Another consideration is how prevalent the condition is that is being treated. If the drug is treating a rare disease, a higher risk of complication may be accepted (these are called orphan diseases because drug companies have sometimes ignored them and there are fewer therapeutic options). If the condition is a common one and the therapy is being used by a large number of people, fewer risks will be acceptable.

Clinical diagnostic tests also carry risk. We will see in chapter 7 that the developers of all diagnostic tests and screening examinations have to decide on an action threshold: the test result that is considered to be "suspicious" or "positive." It is typically a point on a continuous measure, such as blood pressure reading, cholesterol level, glucose level, iron level, or the size of a tumor as observed from a mammogram or lung spirometry test. There is intrinsic risk in testing if the action level is set too high, failing to detect some people who have the disease. Setting too low a level, however, may send many people who do not have the condition for further testing, incurring greater expense, a possibly harmful confirmatory procedure, or unnecessary treatment.

Screening is an area with another type of delineation in risk, that between the individual and the public. The question as to whether mammography should be performed in middle-aged women (the debate is often about women aged 40 to 50) is highly controversial. Personal reports from women who had a mammography that detected a real cancer and so saved their lives are contrasted with the formal evidence that finds no discernable effect of mammography in reducing mortality from breast cancer in this age group. The reasons for this apparent discrepancy are discussed in chapter 7, but this represents a clash between personal risk reduction owed to the screening test and the public health risks and benefits when millions of women are being screened. This is an inherent conflict in all screening and testing programs and often leads to arguments between doctors and their patients with health system managers and planners, particularly among those with the good fortune to live in a country with an efficiently managed and publicly financed health care system.

Risk as an Environmental Construct

Risk is also inherent in setting guidelines for environmental exposures: what is the proper standard for a safe level of ozone or nitrogen dioxide in the air, and is there a reasonable level of dioxide, ionizing radiation, or radon exposure that is safe? In the United States, the leading arbiter for regulating environmental exposure is the Environmental Protection Agency (EPA), and its job is not an easy one. Setting environmental levels too high risks public exposure to potentially harmful substances, but making them too low poses challenges for cleanup. Requiring industry to make "cleaner" (now often, and incorrectly, represented as "greener") products may make consumer products too expensive. We all enjoy the convenience of our automobiles but would object to paying a lot more money for them to have totally clean emissions. Of course, every industry has used this argument many times to fight increased regulation and the expense needed to meet higher standards. However, the case for any standard must be based on sound risk analysis, and the standard must be open to revision as the scientific evidence evolves. Some standards, for example, for dioxin, have been set at unnecessarily low levels and without any evidence that the exposure being regulated leads to harmful effects in people.

Dioxin is perhaps best known as Agent Orange, an herbicide chemical used extensively in the Vietnam War as a defoliant, but it is also widespread in our environment as a byproduct of chemical and pesticide manufacturing and waste incineration. In 1985 the EPA considered dioxin to be a "probable human carcinogen," revised in 2003 as "carcinogenic to humans," and most recently it has been suggested the language should be "likely to be carcinogenic to humans," which, to non-bureaucrats, would seem to be identical to the 1985 classification. The equivocation reflects the uncertainty of the scientific evidence for the safety of dioxin at the low levels normally found in the environment and the need to make assumptions in developing safety guidelines for environmental exposure. In assessing the EPA report, a National Academy of Science (NAS) committee was critical of the EPA analysis on several grounds and suggested the agency had overestimated the human cancer risk.[14] There were two primary problems with the EPA estimation. First, the actual evidence for health risks from environmental dioxin is derived from studies in exposed workers or animals, where the doses of dioxin are many times higher than those experienced by the general population. To arrive at a risk estimate for the lower, unstudied, doses the EPA used a downward linear extrapolation from the risk at the higher doses, assuming the same proportional risk at all levels of exposure. The NAS criticized the assumptions that risk simply decreased proportionally and said data were available to support a "nonlinear" reduction in risk (for example, compared to a higher dose of dioxin, the dose may be 10 percent lower but the risk is 50 percent lower). The assumption of linearity would produce higher risk estimates for usual environmental exposure than a nonlinear reduction in risk. Second, the point where the experimental evidence for adverse health effects from actual doses stops and extrapolation of harm from lower doses begins is called the "point of departure" dose. Where this departure dose is positioned determines the accuracy of the estimated risks from lower doses. The EPA was criticized for not justifying with adequate science the 1 percent cutoff that it used. If the risk estimation at the 5 percent dose level is robust but at the 1 percent level quite imprecise, then estimations below 5 percent will be more reliable than those using the 1 percent departure dose.

Testing is increasingly being conducted to identify genetic variations that may influence risk for future health. A saliva sample and cheek scrapings are mailed to a testing company that, for a not inconsiderable sum, will tell you your risk status. With a few exceptions, these are not very helpful tests. If a woman is found to be positive for one of two breast cancer genes, associated with the familial form of the disease, then a discussion with her doctor is clearly warranted. But for most conditions, such as Alzheimer's, prostate cancer, diabetes, asthma, and cardiovascular disease, the increased risk identified by a genetic test is so small that it offers little meaningful guidance for a course of action. Indeed, for many of these conditions there is no evidence-based remediation that can be recommended. It was the hope of many working in the genetic field that some gene variants would show quite large increased risks, but with a few exceptions this has not materialized. It is now believed that the genetic component of disease causation is due to rare variations in a large number of genes, perhaps for some diseases several dozen or more. For other diseases, different variations in a single gene may increase risk. In this model of genetic causation, determining the increased risk of disease from any single variant becomes extremely difficult to calculate.

Risk is sometimes assessed in terms of how frequently an event is likely to occur. We have the 100-year storm or, as reported recently, the risk of a core meltdown in reactor number 1 at the Three Mile Island nuclear plant in Pennsylvania would be once every 2,227 years (reactor number 2, at the same plant, had a partial core meltdown in 1979). The difficulty with this type of risk estimate is that it is reported with such apparent precision that the public is misled into thinking they are highly accurate. But they are rarely reported with any estimate of certainty (the confidence interval used for a relative risk is one measure of certainty). Even if the estimates were accurate, they leave the impression that the next event will occur 2,227 years from the time of estimation. We conveniently forget that the 100-year storm could happen tomorrow and then not again for a 100 years. This type of risk estimate does not tell us when in the future the event is likely to happen; it is really just a measure of the size of the risk. A core melt down was reported as being expected every 833,000 years at the Quad Cities plant in Illinois, which tells us that the plant is safer than the one at Three Mile Island. It does not tell us when to expect the next meltdown. Yet another problem with these risk estimates is not being certain whether the risk models included all the factors that put the plant at risk. It is most likely that they have not; for example, some nuclear plants have been found to be sitting on geological fault lines many years after they were built, and in this regard the risk estimates must be considered too generous.

This is not to say that nuclear power is a particularly risky source of energy. When I was a boy growing up in the north of England several hundred coal miners died each year in mining accidents, and it is presently estimated by the China Mining Ministry that 6,000 coal miners die annually in that country. Similarly, many people die while working in the oil industry and the United States EPA estimates that 10,000 people die prematurely every year from the effects of breathing air contaminated by coal-burning power plants. No fossil fuel energy sources are free of risk, and deaths from them are greater than those due to the nuclear power industry. Until solar, wind, and other alternate sources of power generation are able to meet all our energy needs, risk profiles would seem to favor nuclear power over more traditional sources of energy.

Our discussion about causality and risk has so far examined the statistical calculations of the association as if they were from a single study. There is little recognition, especially in the earlier writings of Cornfield's era, that replication of findings is important and that data from different studies might be pooled. Nor was adequate attention paid to matters of study validity, including whether bias from such sources as indication, multiple comparison, publication bias, or reverse causality might be operating (described in chapter 6). The fixation with statistical criteria, rather than considering equally important study design and publication factors that influence the validity of observed associations, was not broken until the 1970s.

The concept of risk is always relative to something else; it is always "compared to what." The sailor must decide whether to stay at anchor in a somewhat protected harbor surrounded by rocks or sail into much rougher waters but free from hazardous obstacles. The risk of using a therapy in medicine is compared to using another form of treatment or no treatment at all. The pregnant epileptic woman can be left untreated, incurring potential harm to her fetus from epilepsy itself, or she may be treated with another antiepileptic drug that may not manage her epilepsy as well and incur risks of harm on its own. All vaccines incur some risk but failure to vaccinate carries more. In epidemiology, the number of comparison choices can be great. People who smoke cigarettes may also choose other risky lifestyles. We know they will drink more caffeine and alcohol and will also exhibit other high-risk behavioral factors. Choosing suitable controls to accurately estimate relative risk is far from easy. Should the smoker's controls be free from other risk factors or can that be managed by statistical adjustment? Should the controls be matched so they are as similar as possible to the smokers on other important factors? Should the controls have never ever smoked or smoked, say, less than one or two packs a year? These are all challenges for observational epidemiology, and deciding on criteria for the control group is one of the most important decisions epidemiologists face in designing a study.

The choice of a control group in clinical trials has been the subject of considerable debate. It has been argued that some pharmaceutical company trials carefully select a control group so that the chance of their experimental drug showing benefit is artificially enhanced. Montori and colleagues[15] have described some of the strategies employed, including: various trials sponsored by different drug companies that compared patients using newer second-generation neuroleptic drugs to others in a comparison group using a higher than recommended dose of the older drugs, which is likely to increase the risk of complications in the comparator; or a trial that compared a group using a new antidepressant with a control group taking another drug twice daily, possibly leading to increased daytime sleepiness in the comparator (which would normally be avoided by taking the full daily dose at bedtime); or trials of the efficacy of antifungal agents in patients with cancer, having the comparison patients use an agent administered orally, which reduces its effectiveness; and trials in patients with diabetic nephropathy that used a placebo in the control patients rather than other drugs with demonstrable effectiveness.

We have seen in this chapter that risk is always contrasted to some other exposure or an alternative course of action. When considering risk we should always ask, this risk compares to what? The size of risk, which is itself important evidence as to causality, will depend on what the comparison is.

FOUR

Randomization and Clinical Trials

Do we, holding that the gods exist, deceive ourselves with
unsubstantial dreams and lies, while random careless
chance and change alone control the world?
—*Euripides, 480–406 BCE*

It is appropriate to begin investigating the methods used to demonstrate causality by considering the type of study design that most readily lends itself to doing so. If we wish to determine whether or not a drug therapy or some other type of medical maneuver causes an illness to improve or, alternatively, causes harm, we use a randomized controlled trial (RCT). This study design is often thought of as the gold standard for medical and social research. Here I discuss it as the touchstone against which other research methodologies will be compared. In subsequent chapters I will describe the biases that can arise from a wide variety of sources and to such a degree that they will undermine the credibility of the research, often leading to completely wrong results. The degree to which bias can produce incorrect conclusions is sometimes underestimated even by scientists who spend much of their time trying to reduce its influence.[1] It has been estimated by John Ioannidis, an influential Greek epidemiologist, that up to 96 percent of published research is exaggerated or incorrect.[2] He attributes this to small underpowered studies that by chance cross statistical significance thresholds, multiple analyses of fragile data all amplified by publication bias, and overinterpretation of study results while ignoring potential bias. These problems are all discussed at length in this book.

Randomization is a simple enough concept, but it is not always easy to execute in practice. It allows the play of chance to determine whether someone is treated (the preferred term in medical trials but meaning the same as "exposed," a term we will use for many other research designs) with one type of therapy versus another form of treatment or with no treatment at all. If the randomization procedures are effective, then the group of patients treated with one therapy should be identical to the patients in the other group *in every respect* other than the randomized treatments. Only if the two groups of patients are equivalent can we conclude that any subsequent differences between them result from the treatment used. We can then owe any differences in recovery from illness or occurrence of complications (sometimes called side effects) to the influence of the treatment to which they were randomized. If the differences are sufficiently robust, we can conclude that the treatment *caused* the improvement in the patient's condition or caused any complication.

A Brief History of Randomization

The straightforward structure of the randomized trial makes it the most powerful methodology available to us for studying the effectiveness and safety of medical therapies. It is of interest to ask how early in our history did it become a method for testing the efficacy of medical interventions. The answer, at least as far as is presently known, is that the concept is a surprisingly recent innovation. The Eurocentric view has long held that James Lind conducted the first randomized experiment on board HMS *Salisbury* in 1747 to test various treatments for scurvy, a disease of great interest to the Royal Navy because in those days it killed many more sailors than died from battle. It is not clear how Lind allocated the affected sailors to their treatments, and so we do not know it was done in a truly randomized way. We do know the sailors were divided into six pairs; the first pair was given vitriol (sulphuric acid), the second cider, the third vinegar, then either seawater, barley water, or two oranges and a lemon. Within a few days, the sailors who received the oranges and lemon were about their duties and helping take care of the other sailors. Lind's monumental achievement was written up in his book *A treatise of the scurvy* published in 1753; however, for reasons we will discuss later in this book, the navy delayed for half a century before adopting the prophylactic use of citrus fruit.[3]

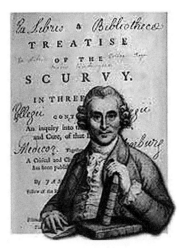

Figure 4.1. James Lind, 1716–1794. Courtesy Sir
Iain Chalmers, James Lind Library.

Lind was not the first to realize that comparing groups of patients who
were treated differently could help deduce whether the treatment was effective and safe. As in so many scientific endeavors, Chinese and Arab scientists
were there first. In China in 1061 CE Ben Cao Tu Jing had two people run
about 2,000 meters, one after being given ginseng while the other person
was not. He reported that only the runner not given the herb had shortness
of breath. Around 900 CE, the Arab physician al-Razi reported in the medical text *Kitab al-Hawi fi al-tibb* that he prevented meningitis in one group
of patients by bleeding them whereas another group of unbled patients contracted the disease. Of course, we cannot conclude from these study designs
that the therapies were effective, but they do illustrate an early understanding of the concept of comparing groups of patients treated differently.

Attempts to discover whether a medical therapy is beneficial and safe by
comparing its use in one group of patients with another treated differently or
not treated at all have not been recorded earlier (at least, no documentation
has been discovered) than the work of al-Razi. Authors of the classical medical text books were remarkably complacent and unquestioning about the
therapies they recommended. Soranus, a Greek and unfortunately named

obstetrician-gynecologist writing in Rome in the second century, appeared very certain about his proscribed therapies (while being so noninterventionist that women delivering under his care and their newborns might have survived the rigors of childbirth better than those treated by any other clinician until the early twentieth century).[4]

This incurious professional view held up to the Renaissance; it was assumed that the Greeks understood everything, and it was only necessary to learn what that was. None of my colleagues who study classical history are aware of any texts describing experimental procedures in the Roman, Greek, or Egyptian periods. We know the Babylonians had a keen interest in chance—but as it related to gambling—and they had a deep knowledge of mathematics (they understood the famous theorem several centuries before Pythagoras). They also studied epidemics (primarily in prisoners and sheep) but appear not to have inquired systematically about their recommended medical therapies. Of course, we cannot be certain that more inquiring minds did not conduct medical studies; our own knowledge is limited by the rarity of ancient manuscripts and tablets, and the evidence for this curiosity may have not survived. There is no doubt as to the intellectual interest of the ancients in other areas of science. It is difficult to believe that such a fundamental aspect of life as maintaining health was not somewhat formally studied until one thousand years into the Common Era. Some scholars see evidence in the Old Testament's book of Daniel for the first documented interest in comparing the effect of an intervention, in this case diet; but even if this were so, it was not conducted in the medical arena.[5]

Sinclair Lewis in his classic novel *Arrowsmith* highlighted some of the difficulties in launching randomized trials in the public arena and showed how the experimental nature of the design can be misunderstood. The protagonist, Dr. Martin Arrowsmith, hoped to test his newly discovered "bacteriophage," which he believed would successfully treat the plague, on a hypothetical quarantined and disease ridden Caribbean island. He proposed to treat half the population with the bacteriophage and then compare its effects on the treated group to the untreated patients. The experiment is never conducted due to enormous opposition from the island's governor, who accuses Arrowsmith of treating the islanders as guinea pigs. Modern medical trialists also face this familiar argument and must cope with the common belief that the experimental treatment must be better than the control. In fact, the majority of trials do not show the experimental drug to be preferable, and results often indicate that it would have been preferable to be in the control group.[6] The ending is particularly bitter for Arrowsmith, whose wife succumbs to the plague.

The First Modern Randomized Trial

In 1948 the *British Medical Journal* published the results of what is now thought of as the first modern trial to incorporate appropriate randomization of patients to the novel therapy and to a comparison (often called control) therapy, as well as other key methodological components of the randomized controlled trial, usually referred to as the RCT. Throughout recorded history tuberculosis has been a major cause of death. In the early twentieth century enormous resources were spent to treat patients with tuberculosis, including building hundreds of hospitals in the United States and Europe. Numerous therapies were tried to manage this disease but with no evident success.[7] In the 1940s the new antibiotic streptomycin became the focus of interest as a possible treatment for tuberculosis. The British Medical Research Council launched a RCT, under the methodological direction of an English scientist named Austin Bradford Hill,[8] which incorporated most of the methodological requirements of the modern RCT.

Eligibility to the trial was restricted to (1) patients with a variety of tuberculosis thought amenable to treatment and (2) those considered to be ineligible for "lung collapse therapy" (although that could be applied if needed). Randomization was "blocked" (the technical term for equalized) in terms of gender and hospital. Patients were allocated to bed rest alone (the usual treatment at that time) or bed rest and streptomycin. Randomization was "confidential" to the treating doctors, and the control patients were unaware that they were in a trial (de facto making this a single blinded trial). All patients were kept in bed for six months and their disease monitored through lung X-ray films examined by three clinicians, two of whom were not connected to the trial. A total of 55 patients entered the streptomycin

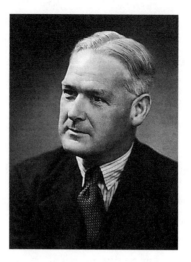

Figure 4.2. Sir Austin Bradford Hill, 1897–1991. Reprinted
from the *Journal of the Royal Statistical Society. Series A (General)*,
vol. 140, Armitage P, A Tribute to Sir Austin Bradford Hill, 127-128.
Copyright 1977, with permission from John Wiley & Sons Ltd.

group and 52 patients the control group. At six months, the results were presented as a percentage (there are no statistical tests anywhere in the paper): 51 percent in the streptomycin group showed considerable improvement versus 8 percent in the controls; the respective death rates were 7 percent and 27 percent. [9] There are aspects of this trial that would not be thought to be the best practice today (for example, most modern trials are double-blinded, meaning neither patients nor treating doctors are aware of the actual therapy being administered although all patients know they are in a trial). However, the streptomycin trial was the first to pay detailed attention to randomly allocating patients to experimental and control therapies, to masking the allocation to the care providers, and to masking the doctors assessing the progress of the disease.

In the following sections of this chapter we review the key features of the modern RCT. The most influential work in codifying the modern construction of RCTs was formulated in two companion papers written in 1976 by Oxford epidemiologist Richard Peto and colleagues in the *British Journal of Cancer.*[10] There are now numerous textbooks devoted to this methodology, which has become an integral part of assessing the effectiveness and safety of pharmaceutical therapies and an essential tool in evaluating public health, educational, and social programs and policies.

In addition to properly allocating subjects to different treatments and best accomplishing true randomization, we must also consider other key sources of bias. Are the treatments "masked" (often called "blinding" in non-ophthalmology trials) to both the patient and the caregivers (this is where the term "double-blinding" originates), is the person assessing the effectiveness of the therapy masked to the therapy, and is a sufficiently large proportion of patients successfully followed up to assess long-term results? We must also consider other important design elements, including whether the analysis is based on randomized patients rather than body parts (unit of analysis error), whether the number of subjects randomized is fully analyzed (intention-to-treat principle), and what the competing risk outcomes are, all of which are discussed below.

Allocation to Treatment (Randomization)

Randomization is without doubt the single most influential design feature of a study which, if done correctly, substantially reduces the opportunity for introducing bias and invalidating the study results. The essential point of randomization is to first create groups of patients who are similar if not identical in all respects. This allows a fair comparison after one group has been treated with the therapy of interest and the other group has been treated in a conventional manner, which may include no treatment. The overriding feature of successful randomization is that it should be masked (this is a different masking from that of the therapeutic intervention, discussed below) in such a way that the treating doctors do not know which treatment the patient was randomized to. This principle leads the investigator to take several practical steps:

1. Avoid randomization until the last moment so as to reduce the chance of a patient being withdrawn from the trial. Doctors

may not favor the selected treatment even when they are guess-
ing what the therapy is. Post-randomization withdrawals are a
major threat to the validity of a RCT and can fatally damage a
trial if there is imbalance in the types of patients entering the
treatment groups.

2. Avoid quasi-randomization strategies that often involve some
   type of alternation; for example, the use of even or odd hospital
   ID numbers, birthdays, or admission days, all of which can produce an expectation of what the patients will be randomized
   to. Even if a doctor guesses incorrectly what the alternating
   therapies are, a bias is introduced if the doctor systematically
   excludes some patients from one of the treatment groups.

3. Randomize at a location that is removed from the treatment
   areas to preclude any knowledge of the randomization reaching the treating doctors. Sealed envelopes are vulnerable to
   high-intensity lamps! The preferred method is to make use of
   24-hour telephone randomization services.

4. Create sequences by generating numbers randomly to allocate
   patients to treatment groups. Often investigators use a "blocking" strategy to ensure an equal number of patients in each
   treatment group after a prespecified number of patients (the
   block size) have been randomized. The block size itself may
   change in a random sequence to further obfuscate the randomization process.[11]

Masking the Therapeutic Maneuver

Masking (or blinding) the therapy to which a patient is assigned has two
primary purposes: (1) it reduces the likelihood that the doctor or the patient
will choose to drop out of the trial and (2) it avoids the chance of a doctor
using an alternative or additional therapy should it be thought that a patient
is being inadequately or ineffectively treated. For example, if a patient or
her doctor knew she was being treated by placebo, the doctor may resort
to other therapies that would result in her no longer being equivalent to

Box 4.1 The First Example of Masking a Treatment, 1800.

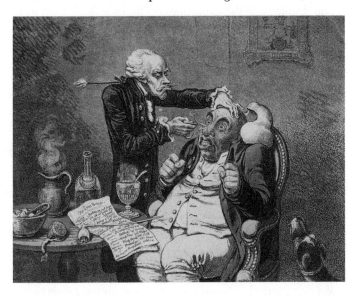

In 1800, Benjamin Perkins, a Yale College graduate living in London, claimed that he could cure numerous conditions with his metallic rods or "tractors" using "electrophysical force." This claim was ridiculed in a cartoon by James Gillray, where a paper lying on the table reads: "Grand exhibition in Leicester Square. Just arrived from America the Rod of Aesculapios. Perkinism in all its glory being a certain Cure for all Disorders. Red Noses, Gouty Toes, Windy Bowels, Broken Legs, Hump Backs. Just discover the grand Secret of the Philosophers Stone with the True Way of turning all metals into Gold. Pro Bono Publico."*

In what may be the first demonstration of masking an intervention to detect a placebo effect, a no-nonsense Yorkshire doctor, Dr. John Haygarth, made a wooden set of "fictitious tractors," painted to look like metal, and in a simple seven-patient crossover study (see chapter 5) comparing the metal and wooden tractors, observed no difference in the effectiveness of either. Masking (or "blinding") is now standard practice in controlled clinical trials. Haygarth published his findings in a pamphlet: *Of the Imagination as a Cause and as a Cure of Disorders of the Body Exemplified by Fictitious Tractors and Epidemical Convulsions*, published in Bath by R. Cruttwell in 1800 (facsimile available at the James Lind Library website).[†]

*Cartoon by James Gillray courtesy of Yale University, Harvey Cushing/John Hay Whitney Medical Library. For a more detailed account of the affair of the metallic tractors, see Booth C. The rod of Aesculapios: John Haygarth (1740–1827) and Perkins's metallic tractors. *J Med Biogr.* 2005;13(3):155–161.
[†]The James Lind Library (http://www.jameslindlibrary.org/), established by Sir Iain Chalmers in 2003, is devoted to understanding the historical efforts made to reduce bias in medical and health research. It is the foremost repository and source of photocopies of original manuscripts and books on the early research in this field.

patients randomized to the experimental therapy. The need to mask often requires innovative methods if the intervention is a procedure other than a drug. For example, in one study nitric oxide gas was being tested to see if it improved respiratory function in preterm babies born with diseased lungs. To mask the therapy being given, identical-looking cylinders were used to administer nitric oxide to the treatment group and to give plain air to the babies in the control group.

In trials using a placebo, the placebo must have the same characteristics as the active drug in its appearance both as a powder and after it is in solution, in its preparation, and in its method of administration. Often the drug "vehicle" (the solution used to dissolve the drug but without the active ingredient) is used. In many modern RCTs, investigators administer two or more active drugs that cannot be masked with the same placebo. In this case a strategy that is called (not eloquently) a "double-dummy" technique is adopted; for example, one drug has to be administered by intravenous infusion and the other by intramuscular injection. In this situation, if two drugs are being studied, one-third of the patients receive one active drug and the other as placebo, another third of patients receive the second active drug with the first as placebo, and the remaining third of patients receive placebo in both administrations. Of course some interventions, such as a surgical maneuver, cannot be masked, and in these cases reliance is placed on masking the person responsible for determining the outcome of the study, which is the subject of the next section.[12]

Masking the Trial Outcome

The third group of RCT participants (after patients and doctors) to be masked to therapy consists of those responsible for assessing the trial "outcome." The most easily measured and least biased outcome is death from any cause. Investigators often use a death registry that is unlikely to be biased (although knowing which therapy a patient had been given may affect how diligently one searches the death records). In assessing death due to a specific cause, the ambiguity of many death certificates requires that this determination be done masked to therapy so as to avoid bias. And for every other clinical outcome — whether a patient's illness or injury has improved, if their mental state is influenced by therapy, or any of a myriad of health indicators that are open to subjective interpretation — it is crucial that this be done without knowledge of which therapy the patient received. In some trials, achieving this objective requires creativity. For example, where a surgical maneuver is compared to a drug intervention, such as comparing the best method for clearing a blocked artery, on follow-up examination all patients may need to be bandaged as if they had received surgery and asked not to inform the examiner what therapy they had received.

Less frequently commented on is the need to mask the data analysts from the actual treatment assignments. When study results are being analyzed, there are many opportunities for introducing bias: how data is being grouped, rounded, categorized, and how missing data is imputed (when a piece of data is missing a value may be assigned based on other information in the dataset). All of these manipulations could be biased if the analyst knew which of the treatment groups was the experimental one and which the control.[13]

How Many Patients Were Followed Up?

If only a small proportion of patients are followed up to assess the study outcomes, the results are unreliable for two reasons. First, there is a chance that the results in the patients not followed may differ from those that are followed to such a degree that the observed study result could be negated or even reversed. Secondly, the reasons that patients are not followed up may be a consequence of the treatment. If patients in one treatment group die more often than those in another group, they may be more difficult (or easy) to follow up; also patients who recover best may move or somehow escape the embrace of the medical care system and be lost to follow-up. Unequal follow-up rates in different treatment groups are a clear sign of a potential bias. Even if the follow-up rates are the same in the treatment groups, it is expected that they include at least 80 percent of those treated, and many trials try for and achieve over 95 percent follow-up rates.

Management Trials and Intent-to-Treat

Imagine conducting a randomized trial to test whether a blocked blood vessel is best treated with a medication or by surgery and the primary outcome of interest is how many patients survive after each procedure. Even in an emergency department, it takes some time to order and prepare medication from the hospital pharmacy, and it may take even longer to have an operating room prepared so that surgery can begin. There will be deaths among patients randomized into the trial before any medication can be given or surgery provided. The question is whether the deaths of patients randomized to these therapies but not yet treated should be counted. It seems obvious that since treatment was not received, they should not be counted, and this is the common answer but it is wrong. Most randomized trials are not simply comparing two types of treatment (medicine or surgery in this example) but rather comparing the *management* of a patient with either of these two therapies. This is a crucial distinction. When a decision is made to manage a patient's care in a certain way, all of the associated problems and ancillary issues become part of the management package. It may take longer to assign an operating room or for a surgeon to start the procedure than it does to prepare and administer a drug. This must be taken into account when comparing therapies. If delayed surgery leads to additional deaths, these must be accounted for to fully understand the mortality resulting from the surgical management plan.

In randomized controlled trials comparing how patients should be managed, the outcomes of all patients randomized to the intended (or planned) treatments need to be counted, not just those actually treated. This is known as the "intent-to treat" principle, and not following it can lead to serious error in interpreting the results of a trial. In our example, if most of the deaths in patients treated by surgery occurred in the time needed to start the procedure rather than by surgery itself, and these deaths are ignored, the results of the trial may incorrectly show that surgery was safer than treatment by medication. Adopting surgery into widespread practice would lead to more deaths not fewer and not necessarily because of the surgical procedure. Bureaucratic delays can cause death as much as the scalpel.

Competing Risks

Another source of error in randomized trials can occur when one trial out-come precludes the occurrence of another. Consider conducting a trial of a new therapy to treat preterm babies who are diagnosed with lung prob-lems. The important study outcomes are survival and bronchopulmonary dysplasia (BPD) that is often assessed at 28 days of life. If the two outcomes are looked at separately, it may appear that with the new therapy BPD is decreased but mortality increased. This is because BPD is being examined only in those babies who survive to 28 days. It is necessary to count the rate of BPD while also accounting for death (an outcome of BPD + death is often used). This problem typically happens when death is an early event so that the second outcome had no opportunity to occur.

The Paradox of Subgroup Analysis

Quite naturally, clinicians are interested in having the patients who are studied in clinical trials match as closely as possible the patients they see in clinical practice. Trials may often cover many age groups, both sexes, patients with a broad range of disease severity and several comorbid or addi-tional conditions. There is strong temptation to slice and dice the data from RCTs to examine whether the overall trial results differ among selected patient subgroups. For example, we may wish to ascertain whether or not women above the age of 50 respond better to the therapy. Herein lies the problem. Most trials have only enough patients to produce statistically reli-able results in the total study group (we return to the delights of statistical power and significance in chapter 8). The point being made here is that as smaller subsets of patients in a trial are studied, the results become increas-ingly unreliable and misleading.

Charles Stein, a Stanford University statistician, described the following paradox: the best prediction of what treatment effect will occur in smaller groups is found in the result from the total study. In our example, the best way to predict the outcome of women over the age of 50 is to look at the overall study result and not at that specific group. (Another study can be conducted for only patients with those characteristics.) Results from small subgroups in a study tend to over- or underestimate the true effect of treatment. Depending on the size of the subgroup and the precision of the overall study result, a correction (Stein called it "shrinkage") needs to be made to estimate the true subgroup effect. There are exceptions: when subgroups are of sufficient interest to be planned in the study protocol, the study can be designed to be large enough to accurately estimate treatment effects in them. A second major problem occurs when analyzing multiple subgroups (for example, studying many different age groups). The more groups that are examined, the more some groups will appear to benefit from treatment (or suffer harm) simply by chance. The problem of multiple comparisons is a very common source of bias in population-based research and will be discussed several times throughout the book. Astrologers rely on this phe-

---

Box 4.2 An Example of the Use of Astrology to Show the Potential for Being Misled by Subgroup Comparisons.

In a reanalysis of the large ISIS2 trial of over 17,000 patients with acute myocardial infarction, which showed a strong overall protective effect of aspirin on mortality ($p < 0.000001$), Rory Collins and colleagues showed that when groups of patients are analyzed within their astrological sign groups, those with the sign of Libra or Gemini did not demonstrate the protective effect. If you believe that astrology can influence health, then you likely stopped reading this book a while back. Otherwise, it will be appreciated that this is a neat demonstration of how subgroup analysis can mislead. If these had been more plausible subgroups, say 12 different blood pressure groups at the start of the trial, some groups might be found where the treatment is ineffective. These patients may be erroneously considered as being unprotected by aspirin, eventually leading to incorrect treatment guidelines. The best predictor of the protective effect in each group is the more robust overall effect.*

*Collins R, Peto R, Gray R, Parish S. Large-scale randomized evidence: trials and overviews. In Maynard A, Chalmers I, eds. *Non-random reflections: on health services research: on the 25th anniversary of Archie Cochrane's Effectiveness and Efficiency.* BMJ Publishing Group, 1997:204.

nomenon for their apparent success because 12 astrological sign groups are given a reasonably broad set of prophecies to millions of people every day. No surprise, then, when a number of these forecasts turn out to be true for a particular person.

The United States Food and Drug Administration (FDA) is properly skeptical about subgroup analyses. In 2005 a federal advisory panel to the FDA recommended that they not approve Xinlay, a possible prostate cancer therapy. They did not trust the study results as they showed effectiveness only in a subgroup of men with advanced stages of the disease and only those who were selected for special analysis after the trial was over. At the same time, Tarceva was recommended for approval as a pancreatic cancer therapy even though it extended survival for only 12 days compared to placebo; however, it did so in a group of patients prespecified in the study protocol.

Errors in the Unit of Analysis

If a dentist conducts a trial of a new toothpaste in 10 patients and 10 other patients are given the old toothpaste, how would the number of cavities be subsequently analyzed? One creative way would be to count all the teeth (assuming a full adult set), 320 per toothpaste, and to calculate the proportion of teeth with a cavity. Another way is to simply add up the total number of cavities per toothpaste. Both of these methods are incorrect and increase the chance of finding a spurious result. When we count the results of a trial, it is important to observe each finding *independently* of all the others. If one person receiving the new toothpaste happened to have cavities in all his teeth (for genetic or other reasons), he would contribute 32 teeth with cavities to the analysis and that would force the result to favor the old toothpaste. A tooth in one mouth is not independent of the other teeth; they all experience the same food, mouthwash, floss, and other paraphernalia of modern oral hygiene, and they have the same genes. For the same reasons, the cavity in a single tooth is not independent of the others in the same tooth. One way to correctly analyze this trial is to count the number of cavities in each of the 20 mouths and to compare the mean number of cavities per person in those using the new, versus the old, toothpaste. Unit of analysis errors occur

---

Box 4.3 Co-bedding Twins in the Newborn-Care Nursery.

Twins are often born before full term and as a result spend time in the newborn intensive care nursery. There is a belief that twins may thrive better if they are allowed to continue their in utero proximity by being bedded together in the same cot during their nursery stay. In order to test this, twins have been randomized in trials to being either co-bedded together or to being placed in separate cots. One outcome of interest is the rate of growth and another is infant survival, but this is a research design that has opportunities for errors in the unit of analysis. The correct way to analyze this data is to consider the twins as a pair. For assessing neonatal growth, the average growth (perhaps measured as increased weight in grams during the first week of life) of each pair of twins would be calculated. For the mortality outcome and other "categorical" factors, deaths could be assessed as none, one, or two in each pair. This would reflect the average number of deaths per twin pair. An incorrect analysis would be to ignore the twin pairing and simply count the events in each twin as if they were independent of each other. Parenthetically, for twin studies, this would also violate another requirement for analysis—independency of observations, discussed in chapter 6. Currently there is insufficient evidence to support the idea that co-bedding is beneficial to twins.

---

when multiple muscles, limbs, organ parts, cell lines, or repeated events such as transfusions, drug administrations, and eye tests are all added up without recognizing that they are not independent because they are occurring in the same person.

Four Phases of the Clinical Trial

There are four phases of research in which the clinical trial is typically used, and each has a different goal and design. Phase 1 is the first human administration of a new drug or a procedure, without any controls, to identify the safest and usually highest dose of a new therapy. The highest safe dose is determined so that subsequent larger trials will not be jeopardized by having a lower than effective dose. Phase 1 dose-escalation studies usually treat two or three patients at increasingly large doses of the new drug as the safety of each dose is observed until, typically, 20 to 50 patients have been observed. Effectiveness is not considered, but this phase may include metabolic and pharmacologic studies. Phase 1 trials are not randomized although Thomas Chalmers, an early pioneer of evidence-based medicine, suggested that the first use of a new therapy in patients should always be given in a randomized manner. He argued that this was the most ethical way to administer a therapy of uncertain benefit and safety.[14]

An example of the benefit of randomizing patients in the early stages of investigating a new treatment was exemplified when fetal brain cell transplantation was being considered for patients with Parkinson's disease. These patients exhibit a characteristic depletion of dopamine in their brain cells, and the study was to transplant dopaminergic brain cells from fetal cadavers into a patient's brain to see if it stimulated dopamine production. When investigators at Yale's School of Medicine submitted a proposal for performing this operation on a small series of four patients to the Yale Human Investigation Committee, the question posed by the committee was whether there would be a big demand from patients to have this procedure. On learning that this would be the case, the committee asked the investigators to randomize their patients so that each would be given either immediate transplantation or would be in a control group for a year, then given the option for a transplant. The result was a small RCT that provided much more useful data (of some small reductions in symptoms and Parkinson's signs) than would have emerged from a simple case series.[15]

Phase 2 trials are often the first to examine drug efficacy and safety in a randomized design. These may include small homogeneous patient samples, typically 100 to 200, and may compare drug doses and regimens for drug administration. Not infrequently, this phase is dropped and investigators move straight into phase 3 trials.

The Phase 3 trial is often the "definitive" efficacy trial conducted in a homogeneous group of patients with a well-defined intervention (developed in the earlier phases). It also addresses the risk of occurrence of more frequent complications. The number of subjects in this phase range from 200 to 20,000 patients (over 10,000 patients are seen in what are called large simple trials discussed in the next chapter). Phase 3 trials are needed to provide evidence that a therapy is effective and safe before it is adopted into everyday practice. The highest level of evidence that a therapy is effective and safe comes from a meta-analysis of multiple phase 3 trials (chapter 13).

Phase 3 trials provide sufficient evidence that a therapy should be adopted, and regulatory agencies in Europe and the United States base their decisions on whether or not to approve a drug on the results of these trials. The trials are expected to have the methodological rigor discussed above. For many therapies, at least two trials are needed and these are often conducted in Europe and the United States. For some therapies one trial is enough to change practice: the evidence from the first trial may be so compelling that a second trial is deemed unethical. The trial conducted to show that lumpectomy was equally as successful as radical mastectomy in the treatment of breast cancer was done only once. More recently, the trial that demonstrated surgery to remove lymph nodes was not needed in patients receiving radiation for breast cancer was by itself sufficient to change practice. But even the most well-done trial is not always adequate to document complications that may occur with a particular intervention. The complications may be very rare, or they may not have been considered plausible outcomes when the trial was first conceived, or they may not be expected to occur until a long time after therapy, such as a late onset cancer.

Phase 4 is the post-marketing trial, conducted after a drug has received approval for marketing. Sometimes, the FDA or other agency may give approval for a new drug with the proviso that a phase 4 trial be conducted. Not infrequently, the results of phase 4 trials have led to drugs having their FDA approval withdrawn or a pharmaceutical company voluntarily withdrawing its product. This recently occurred with Vioxx, a nonsteroidal anti-inflammatory drug used for treating arthritis, and with Rosiglitazone a glycemic-lowering diabetes drug, both of which have been associated with a rare but increased risk of heart attacks. Phase 4 trials differ from other randomized trials in that physicians prescribe the therapy during routine medical practice. Control patients, who do not take the therapy, are usually taken from the same practice, and an effort is made to make them as much as possible like the treated patients. However, without randomization this can produce crucial differences between the two groups of patients, and all the biases that are found in other types of prospective research (chapter 6) have an opportunity to exert their effect in phase 4 trials.

A distinction must be made between phase 4 trials that are conducted to answer legitimate scientific questions and so-called marketing or "seeding" trials. These latter trials are usually conducted by a pharmaceutical company's marketing division for the sole purpose of encouraging doctors to use their product in preference to that of another company, so as to increase their "market share." These seeding trials are unnecessary and may put patients at unnecessary risk of being inappropriately treated.[16] Unfortunately, it is quite difficult for a person who is invited to participate in a drug company sponsored RCT to know if the trial is addressing an important clinical question or is merely a marketing tool designed to boost sales.

Randomization remains the simplest and most complete strategy for comparing the effectiveness and safety of treatments. Although there are methods for statistically correcting imbalances between treated groups, this can be done only if the balancing factors are measured, and measured precisely. Inadequately measured risk factors leave some residual confounding, and unmeasured risk factors cannot be controlled at all, making it difficult to attribute to the therapy of interest any differences observed between the treatment groups.

In trials, randomization is based on chance—but not completely. A deterministic element is introduced, by blocking, stratification, or minimization, which is needed to keep the overall size of the trial from being unnecessarily large. Simple randomization works perfectly well when very large numbers are involved, less so when the available numbers (perhaps restricted by patients with a particular condition or drug supplies) limit the size of the study. It is the power of randomization that permits conclusions about causality to be drawn with some confidence from results obtained in these study designs. It is a lack of randomization that makes causality, when based on all other research methodologies, such an uncertain proposition.

FIVE

More Trials and Some Tribulations

*If one is trying to decide how millions of future patients should
be treated it may often be appropriate to randomize at least
many thousands . . . or even tens of thousands.*
—*Colin Baigent and Richard Peto*

Cluster Trials

Sometimes a traditional clinical trial, the kind discussed in the previous
chapter, where patients are individually randomized to one treatment or
another, will not work. If patients discuss their experimental treatment with
other patients who are in the control group, the latter may then demand to
be treated with the "new" treatment. Similarly doctors, on learning about
a trial being run in their hospital, may prematurely adopt the experimental
therapy making it impossible for their patients to join the trial. In fact, the
majority of trials do not show benefit from the experimental therapy, and
rushing to adopt the new drug may not be beneficial to patients; furthermore, if the trial has to be abandoned because no one can be recruited to
join it, there is no possible benefit to future patients. Bringing trials to a successful conclusion and validating a beneficial therapy, or a non-beneficial
or even a harmful one, is the only way medicine can advance. If these are
likely problems with an individually randomized trial, then a cluster trial
may be an appropriate design (not to be confused with disease clusters, discussed in chapter 9). This is a trial design where an entire hospital, clinic,
village, or even community is randomly selected so it can be treated in the
experimental manner, and another hospital or community is selected to
provide the control group. The number of experimental and control clusters is usually evenly balanced and ranges from one to several dozen in each
trial.

Cluster trials were anticipated by the French philosopher Ernest Renan (1823–92) although since he never mentioned randomization, he was perhaps more interested in the ineffectiveness of prayer than making any methodological comment. He wrote in his *Dialogues Philosophiques*: "In a time of drought, twenty or thirty parishes in the same region would have processions to bring on rain; twenty or thirty would have none. By keeping careful records and by working with a large number of cases, it would be easy to see whether the processions had any effect—whether the parishes which organized processions were more blessed than the others, and whether the quantity of rain with which they were blessed was proportional to their fervor."[1]

A cluster trial was considered to be the study design of choice when colleagues and I were investigating how to promote the more rapid use of surfactant into hospital delivery rooms. This drug was shown in many studies to help expand and maintain the lungs of preterm babies. Not only had surfactant been shown to substantially reduce mortality from lung disease, a common problem in these small newborns, but it worked better if given in the delivery room as soon as possible after the child started to breathe rather than waiting to see if the newborn actually had lung disease. It might have been possible to try to educate a randomly selected group of neonatologists at any one hospital into encouraging earlier use of surfactant, but clearly the risk of new information crossing over to other doctors, in the control group in the same hospital, would be very high. Consequently, we decided to randomize hospitals: all the doctors in any one hospital would either be in the experimental group trying to encourage earlier surfactant use or be a control without such encouragement.

We were privileged to have Jeffrey Horbar, a heavily bearded neonatologist from the University of Vermont, leading our research team. Horbar has a penchant for statistics and evidence-based medicine, and he is also the director of the Oxford-Vermont Network. This network, which includes almost all the newborn intensive care units in the United States and some in Europe, is in many ways a model for how voluntary collaborations among clinicians with similar expertise and responsibilities can foster high-quality research and improved patient care. From the network, we recruited 114 hospitals to join the trial. We randomly allocated them to one of two groups of hospitals: one the experimental group and the other the control.

Neonatologists from the experimental group were invited to a meeting at which they were shown the evidence from meta-analyses supporting the benefit of giving preterm babies surfactant during their first breaths in the delivery room. They were informed of ways in which changes in clinical practice could be made in their hospitals (a methodology called multifaceted collaborative quality improvement, the details of which need not concern us here). The hospital teams were provided with data showing the rates of delivery room surfactant in their own institutions and asked to set their own goals for improvement over the coming months. In addition, an electronic network server was created to facilitate additional communication among the experimental hospitals. The hospitals in the control group received none of this information and continued to practice in their usual way. The primary goal of this type of trial is to observe whether a change occurs in clinical practice. At the end of this trial, surfactant was over five times more likely to be given in the delivery room of the experimental hospitals compared with control hospitals, providing strong evidence to support this type of quality improvement process for improving medical care.[2]

Cluster trials have been used to randomize African villages to assess the success of health education programs for preventing HIV infection and reducing partner violence. Schools have been randomized to study cycle helmet promotion programs, and doctors' offices randomized to examine exercise programs for the elderly. Nutrition programs have been evaluated in clusters of maternity wards in Nepal and in churches and supermarkets. These trials are not as easy to conduct as traditional trials; many people and institutions have to agree to participate and follow the trial protocol, but cluster trials can provide valid answers to important questions when done properly.

Trials That Cross Over

One may ask why not put a patient on one drug, watch her reaction, and then put her on another drug and watch some more? There are several reasons why this is difficult. Once the disease has been treated by one drug there may be some recovery so that the second drug is not treating as severe a condition. Of course, the first drug may have made the disease worse, but the problem with using a second drug remains the same: we cannot fairly compare their effectiveness. However, some conditions can be studied in this way: diseases that are of short duration and reoccur, such as a skin rash, colds, and flu, or conditions that remain constant for long periods of time, like chronic migraines and some mental illnesses. For these types of illness, a crossover randomized trial is not only possible but has several advantages

Box 5.1. The Two Richards.

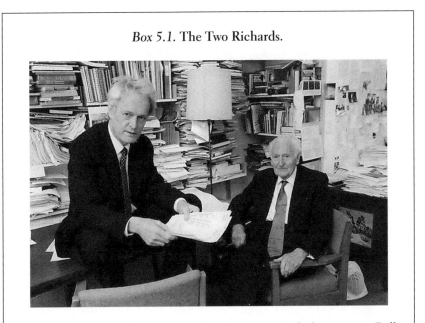

Sir Richard Peto and Sir Richard Doll (1912–2005) in Oxford circa 2000. Doll is considered the foremost epidemiologist of the second half of the twentieth century. He made numerous contributions to observational epidemiology and is especially noted for his early research on smoking and lung cancer as well as extensive studies on the health effects of radiation. Peto, who was trained by Doll, has made major contributions into the statistical analysis of epidemiologic data and the design of randomized trials. He designed and conducted some of the first large simple trials and contributed substantially to the development of methods for meta-analysis (chapter 13). The clutter in Peto's office is quite typical of epidemiologists everywhere.

Photograph by Rob Judges.

over the traditional RCT. As every patient receives both therapies, smaller numbers of people are required in a study. Most important, the variation (some people call it background noise) between study subjects that occurs when some subjects receive one drug and another group of subjects receive a different one is avoided. Problems can occur in crossover trials if too little time passes between the first drug ending and the second one starting. This allows some of the effects of the first drug to carry over to the second period. A "washout period," when no treatments are given, is usually designed into the study. The typical statistical analysis of trials requires some adjusting in this design but despite these problems, the crossover trial offers strong advantages when it is used appropriately.[3]

None of us like having a tooth extracted, especially an impacted wisdom tooth, but relief may be on the way from the Fourth Military Medical University in China. In a creative crossover trial, a portable video eyewear entertainment system was added to the usual nitrous oxide oxygen sedation used in China for the procedure. When the molar tooth on one side was removed the entertainment system was added. On a second visit, for removal of the other molar, the entertainment system was not used. A very large majority of the 38 study patients studied preferred the addition of the video entertainment. Not a surprising result perhaps, but all credit to these dentists and anesthesiologists who put the idea into a formal test with a crossover design.[4]

Large Simple Trials

In the mid-1980s it became clear that many randomized trials were compromised by being so complex that their protocols (the formal document that describe the planned study design and procedures) became very difficult to follow. They also were too small: trials were being designed that were only of sufficient size to identify substantial improvements from therapy. Small or even modest but nonetheless important benefits could be missed, but detecting smaller but real benefits from a therapy requires many more study subjects. The statistical power of a trial is primarily based on how many events, like a death or a cure, are expected under normal circumstances, as reflected by the control group rates and by the number of events expected in the experimental group after treatment, the difference being called the *treatment effect*. When a trial actually starts, it is not unusual for the number of events in the control group to be fewer than anticipated, seriously undermining the planned power of the trial to document a treatment benefit. It is more realistic to expect that many new treatments being investigated will confer only modest benefit, which also requires large numbers of patients in a trial to document an effect.

When a trial is being planned it often undergoes a "Christmas tree ornament" effect. Every collaborator on the investigating team decides that his particular interest—be it a particular type of patient, a variation on the treatment, or additional clinical measures—needs to be included and hung on the trial. However, complicated eligibility criteria and consent procedures for entering the trial can discourage many potential participants. Common yet unnecessary additions to a trial protocol are measurements to try and understand how the treatment may work on a biological level, which may require detailed examinations and uncomfortable invasive procedures that can be highly detrimental to the successful conclusion of a trial. Types of study other than RCTs are needed to answer questions about *why* a therapy may work. The fundamental question for a trial is: does the drug work and is it safe? Some trials find patient recruitment so difficult that the trial has to continue for longer than planned. Indeed, they may go on for such a long time that the therapy being studied is no longer of interest, having been surpassed by newer therapeutic advances.

Richard Peto and Colin Baigent were two of the first researchers to propose a different type of trial to address some of these problems. As they put it, "If one is trying to decide how millions of future patients should be treated it may often be appropriate to randomize at least many thousands . . . or even tens of thousands."[5] These trials, what we now call large simple trials, are characterized by including large numbers of subjects, often up to 20,000 or more participants, and they are designed to answer the principal trial questions of therapeutic efficacy and safety as efficiently and quickly as possible. A large simple trial can detect relatively small but real improvements from a therapy. When multiplied by the large number of patients that need to be treated for the condition, this can result in a substantial degree of public benefit.

The essential features of large simple trials are: avoid random error (chance) by using large numbers of patients, detect small or moderate (but important) effects, study only the most important clinical outcomes, use the uncertainty principle to simplify entry criteria, simplify data collection to what is necessary to answer the primary question, and analyze by intent-to-treat.[6] The "uncertainty principle" criteria for entry to the trial is described simply as: "A patient can be entered if, and only if, the responsible clinician is substantially uncertain which of the trial treatments would be most appropriate for that particular patient. A patient would not be entered if the responsible clinician or the patient are for any medical or nonmedical reasons reasonably certain that one of the treatments that might be allocated would be inappropriate for this particular individual (in comparison with either or some other treatment that could be offered to the patient in or outside the trial)."[7] Importantly, this principle invokes the notion of the clinicians making reasonable judgments of appropriateness, rather than depending on detailed clinical examinations and using sets of predefined criteria that slow down entry into the trial and are unlikely to mimic how decisions will be made to treat patients after the trial is over, should the therapy prove effective.

One of the earliest simple trials, the Chinese Acute Stroke Trial (CAST), randomized 21,106 patients with a suspected acute ischemic stroke in 413 Chinese hospitals. This was a parallel design with patients either receiving aspirin or a placebo. The primary result, death after four weeks, was 3.9 percent in the placebo group and 3.3 percent among those receiving aspirin. This may seem like a small difference, and it would not have been detected with any statistical certainty in a smaller trial, but when combined with another large trial (International Stroke Trial, IST), the case fatality reduction is 900 deaths per 100,000 cases. In China alone, which has some 15 million deaths from stroke over a decade, aspirin would prevent 90,000 deaths in the next decade. It is not unreasonable to think in terms of decades for a therapy because once established a successful therapy is unlikely to be replaced for at least ten years.[8] The CAST trial shows the importance of detecting small but real differences in the effectiveness of a therapy that is used in hundreds of thousands of patients.

Several years ago, I participated in discussions to design a trial to study the use of a steroid drug, methylprednisolone, in the treatment of head injury. At that time, and even now, despite decades of research there is no evidence-based therapy that has been widely adopted for this not uncommon injury. When the CRASH trial (an imaginative acronym for Corticosteroid Randomization after Significant Head injury) was being planned, many different kinds of steroids were being used, although the evidence for doing so was very marginal (many very small trials with inconclusive results). Based on some encouraging results from trials using steroids for acute spinal cord injury, it was thought reasonable and timely to launch a major trial of steroid use to treat head injury. The design of choice was a large simple international double-blinded trial in which 20,000 patients would be randomized to receive steroid or placebo. The CRASH trial had a protocol that was easy to follow and used the uncertainty principle for deciding patient eligibility. The trial was stopped early after recruiting 10,000 patients because of observed higher mortality in the steroid-treated patients. This trial provided valuable evidence against the fairly widespread use of steroids for head injury and became a model for how these types of trials, performed in emergency trauma settings, should be conducted.[9]

Very large randomized trials offer more security against bias and give more precise estimates of increased or reduced risk, particularly identifying effects that are small but consequential when the high prevalence of the condition being treated is considered. In contrast, the same is not true for very large nonexperimental (observational) studies. Many large-scale population based studies have been established to try and understand the very early origins of diseases that occur in adults, and many cohorts have 100,000 subjects or more. Importantly, their large size does not in any way reduce bias. The press, the public, and some scientists are overly enamored with large observational studies. They appear to not appreciate that the risk estimates they produce, which have the appearance of greater precision (accuracy), can be fatally flawed through bias. These large observational cohorts produce the most dangerous type of result: they appear to be precise but they are wrong. This will be discussed more in the next chapter on studying harm.

Factorial Designs

In 1982, I had the privilege of being invited to China to work with some superb epidemiologists from the United States National Cancer Institute in advising the Chinese government on setting up several cancer studies. At that time, China was an ideal place to do cancer research; the prevalence rates of many cancers were considerably higher than in the West, and the absolute number of cases arising from such a large population permitted studies of a size unimaginable elsewhere. Moreover, in the years following the Cultural Revolution, the Chinese people were compliant subjects, whether willingly or not was never certain, and research protocols were followed almost perfectly. One study in Linxian County in Hunan Province tested strategies for the prevention of esophageal and stomach cancer, which occurred at rates up to 30 times greater than in the United States. The area was also known to have substantial nutritional deficiencies, and this became the focus of the intervention.

Almost 30,000 individuals, aged 40 to 69, were studied from four communes in Linxian and randomly placed into four nutritional supplement groups: (1) retinol and zinc, (2) riboflavin and niacin, (3) vitamin C and molybdenum, and (4) beta carotene, vitamin E, and selenium. The trial employed a factorial design that allowed the study to test which, if any, of these different combinations of nutrients was effective. The supplements were given in a large red pill, more suitable for a horse medication, which I was concerned would lead to poor compliance by study participants. The commune leaders, a tough group of veterans from the Long March and still wearing their blue Mao hats and jackets, assured us that compliance was not a problem. They had assigned 300 barefoot doctors to the project to ensure the pills were taken! Over a five-year period, there was some evidence for a decline in death from stomach cancer among those in treatment group 4, suggesting a possible role for nutrient supplementation in this population.[10]

The factorial design is particularly useful when two experimental drugs are being tested and when, in addition to testing the effectiveness of each drug, there is optimism that the two drugs combined may offer further benefit. Because both drugs and the additional (called an interaction) effect can be studied in one trial, these designs can save considerable expense and time and so are used whenever possible. Sometimes, however, factorial trials are not appropriate, and a more traditional trial has to be conducted that randomizes patients into, say, three parallel arms: drug 1, drug 2, and placebo. Several years ago, colleagues and I conducted a trial to see if two drugs, methylprednisolone or naloxone, compared to placebo, when given to patients who were paralyzed following spinal cord injury, would result in improved functional outcomes. In this trial the two drugs had to be given separately because when they had been tested in combination in animal experiments, the cats experienced high mortality, making a factorial-designed human trial inappropriate. We conducted a three-arm trial with each active drug tested against placebo. The trial provided evidence that methylprednisolone could offer modest functional improvement if delivered within eight hours of the injury.[11]

Investigators used a factorial design for the iconic ISIS2 trial, a large simple trial that compared the effectiveness of (1) intravenous streptokinase given for one hour, (2) aspirin taken for one month, and (3) both against (4) placebo, in over 17,000 patients with a suspected myocardial infarction. It used minimization methods (the next section has details) to help balance randomization and combined the large simple trial with a factorial design.[12] The factorial design allowed the separate effects of streptokinase and aspirin to be studied and also if additional benefit was gained by giving patients the combined therapy. In essence, a quarter of the patients each received only streptokinase, only aspirin, both, or neither. The results showed that each therapy was effective in reducing mortality and that giving both therapies together provided added benefit. Impressively, these results persisted for ten years after treating the initial myocardial infarction. This type of large, well-conducted study (over 83 percent of patients were followed up even at ten years) has a profound influence on how patients are treated.

Minimization

It has been said that the generation of random numbers is too important to be left to chance, and indeed there are situations where it is necessary to harness randomization to keep it from running amok. Even the largest trials take their patients from single hospitals, clinics, or local areas, and the number from any one location may be quite small. It is necessary to ensure that they and other planned subgroups have a balanced randomization. It is particularly important to balance the number of patients from any one hospital so that they are fairly evenly divided among treatment groups. Patients from some hospitals may have a more severe form of a disease than those from other hospitals; also hospitals can treat their patients differently in many ways. It is important to ensure that if any differences are seen between treatments, it is due to the treatment and does not result from an imbalance in the hospitals where the patients were treated. When small numbers of patients from any one hospital are recruited, simple randomization can often become unbalanced.

If hospitals were the only concern, then the randomization could be simply "blocked" within each hospital to guarantee equal numbers of patients in each treatment. But there may be several important factors that need to be kept in balance. Blocking on all of them makes randomization very difficult, risks unmasking the trial, and has negative effects on how the data are analyzed. In 1974 Donald Taves, a statistician from the University of Washington, published an important paper proposing a new methodology for assigning patients to trials. He called the method "minimization," and it is now widely used; indeed, many scientists believe it should be uniformly adopted for all trials.[13]

Minimization was not possible before the advent of high-powered computers as it uses a complex algorithm to assign patients to a trial; nonetheless, the concept is straightforward. Here is how it works: suppose we are studying in a multicenter clinical trial whether a drug (D) or surgery (S) is preferable for treating a blocked artery. In each participating hospital we want to make sure the two treatment groups are balanced on some important factors, such as age, obesity, and gender. The first few patients entering the trial are simply randomized, but as the trial goes on, let us say by chance a larger proportion of younger patients are randomized to D and older patients to S. To return to a more even distribution, the next patients entering the trial, if they are young, might be given a 70 percent chance of being randomized to S. Over time, this will equalize the two treatment groups on age. Perhaps the patient's obesity also goes out of balance in the randomization, with more obese patients being treated by S; this too can be corrected by increasing the probability of the next eligible obese patient being randomized to D. Computer programs can now handle minimization on quite a large number of factors resulting in very nicely balanced treatment groups. All of this is done "behind the scenes" with trial investigators unaware of how individual patients are being randomized. A number of variations on minimization have been developed since Taves's original work, but they all have the same purpose of adding, when needed, a deterministic element to the randomization process. Importantly, there is always some proportion of simple randomization left in the algorithm so that no patient is automatically put into one treatment group over another.

Evaluating the Ethics Police

In the last 40 years a formidable force has arisen with the purported goal of protecting the subjects of medical research from harm. In my own university, a process that was managed by one committee now requires four, and the once small support staff of two has grown into a substantial department. There has been a huge increase in regulation at all levels. Consent forms, over which ethics committees spend hours dotting i's and crossing t's, have grown from one page to up to eight or more pages. Now consent booklets are used, which are so large that they require a summary so the patient can read at leisure what commitment she is being asked to make. It can take investigators more than a year to have their protocols approved by all the hospitals needed to participate in large studies. Furthermore, the federal requirements for data security are now so onerous that they require specialized consultants to understand and implement them. University information technology groups have to devote months of time trying to understand ambiguous and ever-changing requirements, and dedicated computers and servers must be employed, resulting in costs of tens of thousands of dollars on a study before the research actually begins. It is reasonable to ask if there is any evidence that research subjects have actually benefited from all of this?

As mentioned above, colleagues and I conducted a trial to see if drugs given to patients suffering an acute spinal cord injury would help them with improved return of function.[14] We proposed that the sooner patients were treated, the better the chance the drug would be effective, and such proved to be the case. Only patients treated within eight hours of their injury benefited from the drug therapy, but only half the patients entering the trial were actually treated within this time frame. Ideally, spinal cord patients would be treated with drugs in the ambulance or in the hospital emergency department, and there is no technical reason why this cannot happen. Unfortunately, the ethics committees had insisted that we obtain patient consent to participate in the trial, and if the patient could not give consent (some were unconscious), consent had to be obtained from a relative. But finding a relative in an emergency situation takes time, and time was of the essence. In fact, no patient who was asked to give consent declined to participate in this trial, and it seems reasonable, at least for this kind of emergency treatment study, to waive the consent procedure entirely. It could be argued that fully half the patients in this trial were potentially harmed by the ethics committee guidelines set up to "protect" them.

Others have more precisely documented the effects of delayed drug administration in emergency settings.[15] In the CRASH trial of steroids for head injury, described earlier, it was calculated that initiation of treatment was delayed by 1.2 hours in hospitals requiring written consent from relatives. It is a well-known paradox in clinical research that doctors can treat all their patients with innovative therapies during normal clinical practice without going through a complex consent procedure, but to treat half of them in a trial, consent is mandatory, often resulting in delay and potential increased harm from the injury. In a trial of tranexamic acid to manage bleeding in trauma patients, it was estimated that delaying treatment one hour reduced the benefit of patients benefiting from the trial from 63 percent to 49 percent. The authors concluded that the "consent rituals" resulted in "avoidable mortality and probably morbidity in participants in the trial." These authors make the point that even the Declaration of Helsinki (one of the primary documents governing medical ethics) states that provisions can be made for research to include patients not able to give consent. Furthermore, patients in emergency situations and their relatives, because of the shock and emergency environment in which they find themselves, are never able to give fully informed consent and so delaying treatment is itself unethical.

What is deeply ironical about the dominance of medical ethics over research practice is that while the recognition that poor science is unethical is axiomatic—indeed, ethical committees spend considerable effort scrutinizing the scientific method of protocols—there is almost no research done by ethical committees themselves to understand whether their procedures are preventing or causing harm. It would not be difficult to randomize study subjects to a long versus short consent form, or emergency patients to consent by relatives versus no consent. We could then assess how well patients are informed and what the impact of the "consent ritual" is on patient clinical outcomes. The very limited evidence to date suggests that more harm than good may be being done, at huge institutional cost.

In the 1980s, frozen embryo implantation was being developed to assist couples who had difficulty conceiving. One of the tasks, undertaken by a subcommittee of the ethics committee of which I was a member, was to determine the appropriate number of embryos that should be implanted. Using too few risked none surviving but if too many were implanted, the dangers to the mother of higher-order pregnancies, particularly four or more fetuses, was significant. After much discussion and review of the (incomplete and inadequate) literature, we concluded that the number of embryos implanted, if memory serves, would be three. In retrospect, this was an inappropriate conclusion. In the face of limited experience and evidence, it would have been more ethical for us to recommend a randomized trial, in which women had two, three, or four embryos transplanted. In the face of uncertainty, this would have been a more ethical approach to treating the individual patient, and it would also have contributed to knowledge. Women in the future would have been given the opportunity to receive more evidence-based treatment. In 2012, a study of 124,148 in vitro fertilization cycles, which resulted in 33,514 live births, recommended avoiding the transfer of more than two embryos and considered that for many women single embryo transfer was preferred.[16]

The importance of double-blinding has spread beyond the realm of testing disease treatments to jurisprudence. The police lineup where a victim or witness is asked to identify the perpetrator of a crime, among four to six "fillers," is a staple of the justice system. Yet in more than three-quarters of the first 183 cases where DNA evidence exonerated convicted persons, incorrect identification by witnesses had been the leading reason for the initial conviction. Witness lineups have several features. They are either simultaneous, in which all the people in the lineup are seen together, or sequential, where they are seen one at a time. Lineups are also live, or they are, more commonly, of photographs. Simultaneous lineups require the witness to compare suspects to each other whereas the sequential lineup requires the witness to depend on comparing each suspect to their memory of the perpetrator. In these circumstances it is usual for the police officers administering the lineup to know who the actual suspect is. Questions have arisen as to whether this provides clues to the witness as to whom the police think the perpetrator is—perhaps by facial expressions, nuances in voice, or language or other subliminal behavior. Double-blind sequential lineup studies are being conducted in which the police officers administering the lineup are themselves "masked" as to the identity of the "real" suspect, but these studies remain controversial. Laboratory studies are relatively easy to conduct but their generalizability to real-life conditions is questionable. Studies done "in the field" are plagued by not always being certain who the real perpetrator is.[17]

In the next chapter, we will leave the reassurance that randomized trials, when they are conducted properly, generally provide valid results that reflect causal associations: that the treatment does cause an improvement in recovery or it does cause complications. We turn to the largest single body of studies in the human research literature, those from observational epidemiology. Investigators who conduct clinical trials have harnessed randomization in a way that substantially strengthens the inferences that can be drawn about causality. In contrast, observational studies can be rendered meaningless, and worse, despite an appearance of rigor, they may provide wrong results. Random occurrences or chance are a major source of bias and, as we shall see, a principal reason why it is so difficult to draw conclusions about causality from observational data.

SIX

Harm

Irrationally held truths may be more harmful than reasoned errors.
— *Thomas Henry Huxley*

It is considered unethical to randomize people to test treatments with the intent to see if exposure to a drug or chemical will cause them harm. Institutional Review Boards (IRBs), the present-day arbiters of ethical research practice, would have shown Goldberger the door if he had gone to them requesting permission to randomize people (let alone prisoners) to a diet that might induce pellagra. Fortunately for him, the prisoners who earned their release from prison, and us, Goldberger did not have to obtain consent from a modern IRB. If the principal goal of a study is to see whether a drug or chemical causes complications, induces pregnancy or birth complications, or increases risk for cancer, autism, Alzheimer's, or any other disease, then the reassurance that is provided by randomization to the exposure, for protecting against bias, must be abandoned.[1] Observational methods of research are required, and these are fraught with potential to mislead. These types of studies often lead to daily headlines in the press and not inconsiderable confusion in the public mind because they often conflict with the results of other similar studies. It is important to review in detail the structure of these studies, how they are subject to bias, and consider what readers of the studies (and even readers of the newspaper reports) should look for to identify the more valid studies from those that are probably wrong.

There are two large classes of observational study: prospective and retrospective, each with inherent variations in methodology that carry the potential for sufficient bias to threaten the validity of their results. The prospective observational study is most similar to a randomized trial, but the exposure occurs during the course of everyday life instead of by randomized allocation. Exposure may result because a doctor prescribed a drug, a chemical is found in the workplace, or due to environmental contamination of one's living space. In prospective designs, investigators follow the exposed study subjects over time to note how many develop the disease of interest. The disease rates are then compared to a group of unexposed people. Many large groups (technically called "cohorts") are followed for years and are studied for many different exposures and a broad variety of health outcome. There have been prospective studies of nurses and doctors and of people who live in selected towns or work in particular industries. These can be very large cohorts, some with up to 100,000 participants; however, the large size should not be assumed (as it often is in the press) to be an unmitigated advantage. Unlike the very large RCTs, where bias is controlled in the design and the large size helps with study precision (increasing confidence that the estimates of benefit and risk are correct), the large observational studies have as much potential for bias as the smaller studies. As we shall see below, they may produce what appears to be a more precise result, but it also may be biased.[2]

Some prospective studies do not literally follow their subjects over time: instead, the cohorts of exposed and unexposed subjects can be constructed retrospectively. For example, researchers may study records available in large national data bases, such as those found in Denmark or Sweden, in the records of health maintenance organizations like Kaiser Permanente, or in databases organized by government agencies like Medicaid. The availability of past exposure data allows the subjects to be "followed" over past time to determine who developed the disease of interest. Sometimes called "historical cohort studies," these designs can produce quite valid results although they too are not free of potential bias, as discussed below.

Retrospective studies are backward-looking, in that a group of people with the disease (traditionally called "cases") are examined to ascertain whether they were exposed to the agent under study. Their exposure rate is compared either to standard population rates or to another group of similar subjects (the controls) who are asked, in what should be an identical manner, about their past exposures. Due to the retrospective nature of the inquiry, the case-control study is the design most fraught with potential bias. However, for investigating rare diseases, it is the only practical study design available to us. For example, if one wanted to study adults with glioma brain tumors to see if exposure to cell phones had increased their risk of cancer, it would take a prospective cohort of two million cell phone users and another two million non–cell phone users to detect with a reliable degree of certainty a threefold or more increased risk of tumors. But in a case-control study, we could detect a similar risk increase with a case group of only 100 glioma patients and the same number in a control group.[3]

The term "bias" has already been introduced and, as we will see below, it comes from many sources. Bias is systematic or random error that leads to an incorrect estimate of the size of association of a risk factor with the occurrence of disease. Association can be defined as a statistical link which is shown in what is called a "2 $\times$ 2" table (box 6.1): the exposure is dichotomized into "exposed" and "not exposed," and the disease similarly split into "disease present" or "not present." All studies can be simplified in this man-

---

Box 6.1 Structure of a Study to Evaluate the Effect of an Environmental Exposure.

	Disease		
	Yes	No	Total
Exposed	a	b	$n1$
Unexposed	c	d	$n0$

Rate in exposed group = $a/n1$

Rate in unexposed group = $c/n0$ Relative Risk (Risk Ratio) (RR) = $\dfrac{a/n1}{c/n0}$

Risk Difference (RD) = $a/n1 - c/n0$

Number Exposed to Produce Harm (NNH) in one person = $1/RD$

Odds Ratio (OR) = $\dfrac{ad}{bc}$

---

ner, and it often helps to understand any research result by looking for its intrinsic 2 × 2 table. In many studies, the exposure will have more than two categories, perhaps representing different doses or exposure levels. This can be very influential for determining if causation has been documented. The disease outcome may also be measured in several categories, for example, to reflect disease severity or the degree of certainty that a disease has been diagnosed. These more complex tables are all variations of the 2 × 2 and will be introduced in more detail later in the book.

Confounding is another concept that must be introduced here. It is a special type of bias that occurs when a factor unrelated to the disease is intimately connected to the exposure and in consequence may be incorrectly linked to the disease. The classic example, taught to all students of epidemiology, will serve well here. Yellow fingers are a common characteristic of cigarette smokers, and so yellow fingers will be more common among patients with lung cancer (we say they are strongly associated with the disease). However, yellow fingers are confounding the disease association, which we know is really linked to cigarette smoking. A less obvious example, and one that for a time misled researchers, linked high caffeine use to an increased risk of myocardial infarction. Perhaps not surprisingly, high caffeine users are also more likely to be smokers, and it is actually smoking that is the causal factor for heart disease. In this example, smoking is confounding the caffeine consumption association. We now turn to some of the more important specific types of bias.[4]

Sources of Bias

Selection Bias

If more exposed people who already have the disease enter a study than do exposed people without the disease, this bias will spuriously increase risk. By the same token, if fewer exposed people with disease participate in studies, then the risk estimates are correspondingly decreased. In general and unsurprisingly, people with diseases are much more likely to participate in research studies, and this bias will usually seem to show increased risk in the study results.

Box 6.2. An Example of How Selection Bias Works to Spuriously Increase Apparent Risk.

Drug exposure rate in all pregnant women = 10 percent.

Assume preeclamptic women who are also drug-exposed are twice as likely to agree to join study as unexposed preeclamptic women. Drug exposure rate = 20 percent.

Healthy women join study with normal drug exposure rate of 10 percent.

Calculated but false increased risk of the drug being associated with preeclampsia = 2.0.

This example shows how selection bias works to spuriously increase apparent risk. Assume that researchers are studying whether women exposed to a particular drug in pregnancy have an increased risk of preeclampsia. The study investigators select a group of women who have had preeclampsia from a hospital, and a control group of women without preeclampsia from the same hospital. They then inquire about the use of the drug during pregnancy. However, the local newspaper has already printed stories of the potential risk from this drug for preeclampsia, and as a result women with preeclampsia who used the drug are more likely to be interested in and agree to join the study than are women who used the drug but had a normal pregnancy. Assume the population rate of drug exposure is 10 percent and that is also the rate of exposure in the women with normal pregnancies who join the study. If women with preeclampsia who used the drug are twice as likely to join the study, the rate of exposure in the preeclampsia group will be 20 percent producing an apparent, but false, twofold increase in risk from the drug.

Studies especially prone to selection bias are those originating in special referral clinics or hospitals where the disease of interest is being treated; registries where participation is *voluntary*, such as some registries that record birth defects or monitor patients who have used certain drugs (for example, the acne treatment Accutane). Other registries prone to selection bias when patients from them enter studies are those registering special therapies, such as assisted reproductive technologies to help fertilization. Some registries, such as for cancer and infectious disease, legally require registration, which helps reduce bias; however, individual subjects may differentially agree to participate in research projects, which could then be susceptible to selection bias.

Disease Ascertainment Bias

When we increase the intensity of a search for disease in persons whom we suspect were exposed to some agent of interest, compared to the search in those not exposed, we incur disease ascertainment bias. Many diseases are difficult to diagnose and any diagnosis may be influenced by the intensity of the search for the signs and symptoms of disease. For example, there may be a more thorough search for a heart malformation (many of which are usually missed at birth) in newborn children known to have been exposed to a drug of interest, which will reveal more disease that artificially inflates risk.

It is implausible to expect that exposed persons will be examined less than unexposed study subjects, so this bias will always work in the direction of overestimating drug risk. In a paper looking at the evidence for Paxil, an antidepressant medication alleged to increase the risk of congenital malformations in the children of mothers who use it while pregnant, the authors comment: "It has been our clinical impression that pregnant women with psychiatric conditions whom we have counseled utilize substantially more diagnostic tests in pregnancy than healthy women. . . . Women receiving SSRIs and, in particular, paroxetine, utilized a mean of 20% to 30% more ultrasound and echocardiogram procedures during pregnancy and more than 2-fold more echocardiograms in the first year of the infant's life when compared with women not using psychotropic drugs."[5]

These tests will assuredly find minor heart malformations that would otherwise be missed in the children not being examined so closely. In another paper on the same topic, the children of women known to have used antidepressants may have been examined more carefully to detect congenital malformations, which then appeared disproportionately more frequently among them. This potential bias was recognized by the study authors, who remarked, "We cannot rule out that surveillance bias may explain at least some of the increased risks in our study."[6]

Ascertainment of Exposure Bias

A paper published in the 1970s led to one of the greatest public health scares of the 1970s and 1980s. The paper reported that children living in homes with a higher than normal exposure to electromagnetic field (EMF) radiation (which is non-ionizing radiation, unlike the ionizing radiation from nuclear reactions which is well known to be able to cause cancer) were at a two to three times increased risk of developing leukemia. The study assessed EMF by measuring the home's proximity to an electric transformer and by the thickness of the wires bringing electricity to the home.[7] However, the measurements of distance and wire thicknesses were imprecise. The interviewers knew which homes belonged to leukemia cases and which to healthy controls. It seems almost certain that this led to overestimation of wire thicknesses and underestimation of distances to transformers in the leukemia cases. The interviewer also asked the mothers about other leukemia risk factors such as exposure to chemicals. Researchers in other studies where the wire-coding assessors made these measurements, not knowing if it was the house of a case or control, found much weaker associations between EMF and leukemia (see figure 6.1).

A meta-analysis of 56 studies did not find evidence to support an association between EMF and leukemia; another meta-analysis of ten studies found no association with childhood brain tumors.[8] It is difficult to ensure that study interviewers do not know whether they are interviewing a case or a control respondent as the cases may be obviously ill or they may be all too willing to discuss their illness with the interviewer. Opportunities for interviewers' bias in recording the exposure status of a research subject are numerous.

Recall Bias

When asked about the past history of drug use, lifestyle behaviors, or chemical exposures, healthy subjects are less likely to remember these experiences and tend to underreport them. Patients with a disease may mentally scru-

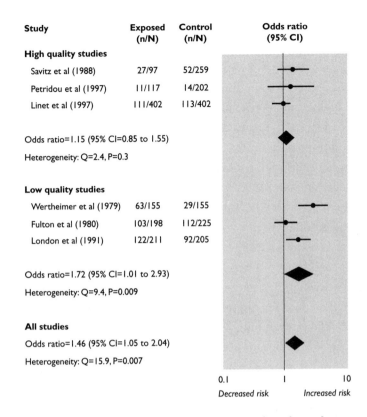

Study	Exposed (n/N)	Control (n/N)	Odds ratio (95% CI)
High quality studies			
Savitz et al (1988)	27/97	52/259	
Petridou et al (1997)	11/117	14/202	
Linet et al (1997)	111/402	113/402	
Odds ratio=1.15 (95% CI=0.85 to 1.55)			
Heterogeneity: Q=2.4, P=0.3			
Low quality studies			
Wertheimer et al (1979)	63/155	29/155	
Fulton et al (1980)	103/198	112/225	
London et al (1991)	122/211	92/205	
Odds ratio=1.72 (95% CI=1.01 to 2.93)			
Heterogeneity: Q=9.4, P=0.009			
All studies			
Odds ratio=1.46 (95% CI=1.05 to 2.04)			
Heterogeneity: Q=15.9, P=0.007			

0.1   1   10

Decreased risk   *Increased risk*

Figure 6.1. Meta-analyses of six case-control studies relating residential exposure to electromagnetic fields to childhood leukaemia. Summary odds ratio calculated by random effects method. Adapted by permission from BMJ Publishing Group Limited. Higgins JPT, Thompson SG, Deeks JJ, Altman DG. Measuring inconsistency in meta-analyses. *BMJ.* 2003;327:557–560. Copyright 2003.

tinize their past history for what may have "caused" their illness, resulting in more accurate recall. Overreporting is unlikely as people rarely lie in an interview by reporting exposures that never existed. But the net result is the same, an apparently greater rate of exposure in people with the disease.

A controversial political as well as scientific topic in the 1970s was the possibility of induced abortions increasing risk for problems in future pregnancies and the mothers' increased risk of suffering depression or other maladies. It was ammunition in the debate about legalized abortion that raged in many countries. Many studies examined whether the risk of breast cancer was increased after an induced abortion, although there was little plausible biological rationale for it. Because breast cancer is a relatively rare disease, researchers used a case-control design and a meta-analysis of these studies is shown in figure 6.2. Immediately apparent is the large number of studies that show an increased risk, an overall 30 percent greater risk for breast cancer after an induced abortion. These data were reported to have figured prominently on the website of the National Cancer Institute during the Reagan presidency.

We now know these studies systematically overestimated the risk, which is actually zero. In 1997, a large study from the national registry in Denmark was reported which linked the medical records of one and a half million women to their abortion history and their diagnosis of breast cancer.[9] There was absolutely no difference in the rate of breast cancer among women who had or did not have a history of a prior induced abortion. Why then the discrepancy with the case-control studies? The record-based studies, which simply linked existing records, required neither an interview nor patient recall, thereby providing no opportunity for recall bias. In contrast, the case-control women were asked in detail about their pregnancies, including induced abortion. It seems apparent that a woman with breast cancer would likely fully report her pregnancy and abortion history (there are well-accepted pregnancy-related risk factors for breast cancer, such as first births at older age). It is also likely that healthy women *underreported* their prior abortions, especially in settings where abortion is not considered socially acceptable. The net result is an underreporting of induced abortion in the control group, more exact reporting in the cases, and the apparent but incorrect result of a history of induced abortion being associated with breast cancer.

Because case subjects recall their drug exposures more accurately than control subjects, risk in cases using a drug is overestimated. It is theoretically possible that patients with a disease would "deny" their exposure, which

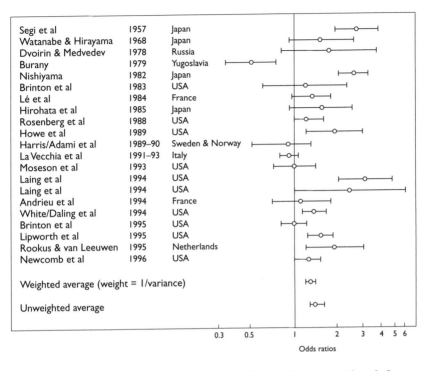

Segi et al	1957	Japan	
Watanabe & Hirayama	1968	Japan	
Dvoirin & Medvedev	1978	Russia	
Burany	1979	Yugoslavia	
Nishiyama	1982	Japan	
Brinton et al	1983	USA	
Lé et al	1984	France	
Hirohata et al	1985	Japan	
Rosenberg et al	1988	USA	
Howe et al	1989	USA	
Harris/Adami et al	1989–90	Sweden & Norway	
La Vecchia et al	1991–93	Italy	
Moseson et al	1993	USA	
Laing et al	1994	USA	
Laing et al	1994	USA	
Andrieu et al	1994	France	
White/Daling et al	1994	USA	
Brinton et al	1995	USA	
Lipworth et al	1995	USA	
Rookus & van Leeuwen	1995	Netherlands	
Newcomb et al	1996	USA	

Weighted average (weight = 1/variance)

Unweighted average

0.3   0.5   1   2   3   4 5 6

Odds ratios

Figure 6.2. Biased association of prior induced abortion with risk for breast cancer. The data suggest an approximately 30 percent increase in risk of breast cancer after a previous induced abortion, but this does not take into account likely substantial underreporting of abortion in the healthy control group. Adapted by permission from BMJ Publishing Group Limited. Brind J, Chinchilli VM, Severs WB, Summy-Long J. Induced abortion as an independent risk factor for breast cancer: a comprehensive review and meta-analysis. *J Epidemiol Community Health.* 1996;50(5):481–496. Copyright 1996.

would underestimate risk, but this has never been observed in studies of recall bias. In some studies, subjects are asked to recall their drug exposures occurring months or years earlier. Not surprisingly, compared to remembering recent events, questions about the distant past have been found to further increase the likelihood of recall bias.

Indication Bias

How can we disentangle the consequences of disease, for example, a higher risk of heart attack, or conditions associated with it (perhaps, smoking, malnutrition, alcohol, obesity), from complications owed to the drug treating it (that is, "indicated" for the disease)? For example, mothers using an antiepileptic drug may have a higher rate of problems in pregnancy; these women may also suffer from other conditions such as anxiety, depression, autism, and attention deficit hyperactivity disorders, all of which may be responsible for the pregnancy complications. When birth complications occur are they due to the drug used to treat the mother's epilepsy or are they due to the epilepsy itself and related conditions?

It is no easy task to separate the effects of diseases from the effect of drugs used to treat the disease as causes of additional complications. For example, when we discuss concepts of causation later in the book, we'll see that drug dose is an important contributor in assessing causation when the risk of disease is observed to increase with greater exposure, such as a higher drug dose. However, even apparent drug dose effects may be caused by indication bias as the more severe disease is treated by higher drug doses. Moreover, if the drug is being used as second line therapy after initial treatment failure, the disease is likely to be more severe in those patients and comparisons with less severely diseased patients may be misleading.

We have seen that in properly designed randomized trials, the only difference between patients in the experimental group and those in the comparison group is use of the drug of interest. In observational studies, there can be many important differences between the two groups, and some of these will not be understood or measured and so cannot be corrected by statistical analysis. The reasons for a doctor prescribing a particular medication or a therapy to one patient but not another is often not recorded. The nuances of prescribing practice are rarely mentioned in studies, but these may result in indication bias. What is it about a patient's medical or physical condition, personal or social situation that makes a doctor choose to prescribe one drug over another, or possibly none at all? For many complex chronic conditions, such as asthma, arthritis, cancer, chronic pain, or depression, a doctor has numerous therapeutic choices. If we seek to evaluate the possible complications of therapies using observational studies, we need to understand the reasons why some prescribing choices are made over others.

Indication bias may also affect the control group. In a study of pancreatic cancer conducted in a Boston hospital, investigators observed that the cancer cases drank three or more cups of coffee two to three times more frequently than the controls, who had been selected from the patients with gastrointestinal (GI) complaints. It was suggested that this reflected a causal association and that coffee use "might account for a substantial proportion of the cases of this disease in the United States."[10] Only later was it appreciated that early symptoms of gastrointestinal disease in the GI control group, probably long before they were hospitalized, would have led them to *reduce* their coffee consumption. The pancreatic cancer patients were not drinking more coffee; it was the control group that was drinking less.

Multiple Comparisons Bias

As discussed throughout this book, there are numerous opportunities for bias, challenging our estimation of risk and chance. The convention in science is that when an association is being examined, there should be 95 percent confidence that the observed estimate of the size of the association is correct and 5 percent chance that it is wrong. If an association meets this criterion, it is said to be "statistically significant" (not to be confused with clinically significant), and it is given special attention as an association that should be studied further. This confidence limit is set high (for example, higher than the law which uses a 51 percent confidence limit, "more likely than not") because it is felt that in science the possibility of making a mistake in accepting an association that is actually false is more damaging than not accepting an association that is real (this second level is often set with 80 percent confidence). These matters are discussed more fully in chapter 8.

Here we are concerned with what happens to these levels of confidence when more than one association is being examined. The more associations we observe, the greater the chance that some of them will be false. If

100 chemicals are studied for their association with a cancer, by chance we expect 5 will meet the conventional standard of statistical significance. In this situation, it is not possible to separate which of the observed associations are due to chance and which may be of real interest. More stringent guidelines are required and these are called "corrections for multiple comparisons."[11]

Almost all studies examine many combinations of exposure with disease, and studying 100 or more associations in a single publication is not uncommon. In recent years genetic studies, which look at 500,000 to 1 million different single-nucleotide polymorphisms (SNPs, see chapter 10 for details) for an association with disease, have highlighted the difficulty arising from multiple comparisons. For example, in the latter case 50,000 SNP associations would occur by chance at the typical 5 percent probability level. Many advances have been made to account for both the multiple observations and the linkage that occurs among SNPs across the genome: blocks of SNPs are linked within genes so that they are dependent on each other; if one is associated with disease others will necessarily be also. Very few nongenetic studies formally correct for multiple comparisons, although many authors caution that their statistically significant results may have been produced by the many associations tested.

Dependent Observation Bias

Statistical methods used to study the causes and treatment of disease usually require that a study subject be entered into the study only once. In risk factor research, using the same people in a study multiple times introduces bias because the observations are no longer independent. This can be a particular problem in studying illness during pregnancy or in children. Let's use an example of a study to test whether a drug for treating nausea in pregnancy is associated with an increased risk for birth defects in the exposed child.

Mothers in a study of a potential teratogen (this is defined as something that causes birth defects) should be counted in the study only once, even if they have had multiple births. This is because some mothers may have an increased risk for having a child with a congenital malformation for reasons unrelated to the drug (for example, because of family history or because she is alcoholic). Her risk of having a child with a malformation in a second pregnancy is biased by her other risk factors and does not fairly test the risk of the drug exposure. Because there is recurring higher risk for malformations in subsequent pregnancies after the birth of one malformed child, this bias increases the chance of observing a spurious higher risk with the drug.

Dependent observation bias also occurs in counting multiple births such as twins. The preferred methodology is to randomly pick one pregnancy, or one birth, to enter into the study. Sometimes studies will pick only the firstborn, but this may introduce bias because first pregnancies differ from other pregnancies in many ways.

For studies of rare diseases, the same patient may be entered into different disease registries, or the hospital where they were treated may enter their data into different databases that are used in a number of studies, so that the same patients are being counted in several published reports. It is also not unusual for doctors to publish reports from hospitals or registries on a continual basis, and thus the original patients are included in subsequent publications of the same data. When this repetition is ignored, it seriously influences the calculated risk estimates when data are pooled for meta-analysis (chapter 13). Many genetic studies make their data publicly available, and here too the same data may be published in multiple reports, which, if unrecognized, leads to problems in meta-analysis.

Confounding and Residual Confounding

Confounding occurs when a factor that may increase disease risk is linked to a second factor that may also increase the risk. Childhood asthma symptoms have been associated with air pollution, but what is the contaminant in the air that actually increases asthma risk? Or, indeed, are there multiple contaminants? Ozone is of special interest, and another component is particulate matter (PM), especially the smaller particles (PM 2.5 microns in diameter or less). These two pollutants are fellow travelers: as one increases or decreases in the air so does the other. In our language of bias, one confounds the other. Even with special statistical methods, it is very difficult to disentangle the independent effects of these confounding exposures on

Box 6.3. Monty Python Confounds.

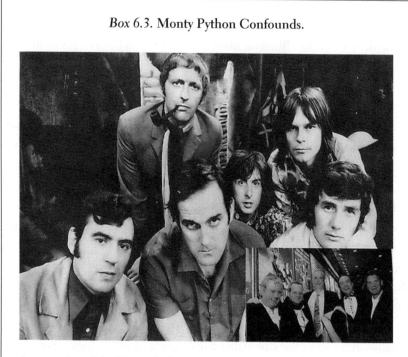

At a reunion of the Monty Python comedy team, which has been praised by the estimable *New York Times* reporter John Burns for its "puncturing of British pomposity, social protocols and pretensions," one member was missing, having died of throat cancer. It was Graham Chapman, seen smoking the pipe in the early photograph. If not being seen with a pipe is assumed to mean the other Pythons didn't use one, the evidence from this picture suggests a strong association between pipe smoking and throat cancer (a ninefold increased risk in the way these are often calculated). However, this would be a premature conclusion as Chapman was also described in his obituary as being a "ruinous alcoholic." This limited evidence for an association between pipe smoking and throat cancer, already based on a small number, one (!), is totally confounded by the second risk factor—alcohol—but this is not unlike many early reports of cases linked to an exposure found in the medical literature. They form very useful hypotheses for future investigation but cannot themselves document a reliable association.

Photo of Monty Python group, 1969, "Flying Circus." Copyright © BBC Photo Library. Monty Python group reunion, 2005, New York City. Courtesy, Lyn Hughes, Lyn Hughes Photography.

asthma symptoms.[12] This is unfortunate when it comes to planning remediation at their source: ozone is a product of power plants, gas stations, and aircraft, whereas PM 2.5 is a product of traffic exhaust, fossil fuels, wildfires, and volcanoes.

Scientists are well aware of the need to control for confounding when studying risk associations, but the confounding factor may be unknown and so may not have been assessed (the great strength of randomization is that it controls for unknown as well as known confounders). Or, the confounding factor may be known but has been inadequately controlled, resulting in residual confounding. For example, smoking is a continuous exposure, as people smoke individual cigarettes not packets of them. In a study of alcohol use and cancer, where smoking is an important confounder, it may be assessed using a dichotomy (smoked: yes/no) or as a categorical variable (none ever / not current smoker / current smoker). This may be inadequate for controlling the confounding effects of smoking because even within the categories, smoking more versus few cigarettes may also influence risk.

One of the many unresolved problems of epidemiology, which continues to fascinate the public and epidemiologists themselves, is whether imbibing wine, particularly the red variety, reduces the risk of various diseases, especially cardiovascular disease. It is also uncertain whether all types of alcohol confer benefit or only wine. An obvious difficulty in this type of research is to control for all the different food choices that the wine drinkers may make compared to those of the non-wine drinkers. This problem was creatively solved by Danish epidemiologist Ditte Johansen and her colleagues; they undertook what might be the first supermarket epidemiology project, reviewing the sales slips from the inventory control data of 3.5 million transactions from 98 Danish supermarkets.[13]

The results of the study are shown in figure 6.3. Compared to beer purchasers, who also enjoyed soft drinks, lamb, and sausage, the wine purchasers were much more likely to buy olives, low-fat cheese, and fruit or vegetables. Many studies have controlled for other lifestyle differences (such as smoking and exercise) between wine drinkers and non-wine drinkers, but it is very difficult to correct for the many more nuanced differences in diet found in people drinking these beverages. Sadly, the health benefits

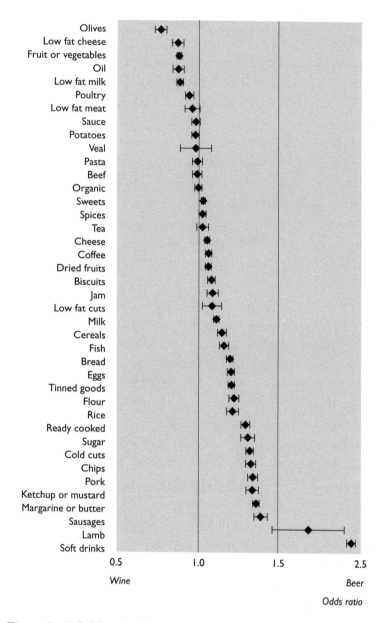

Figure 6.3. Likelihood of beer and wine buyers buying items of food. Items with an odds ratio lower than 1 are bought more often by wine buyers and items with an odds ratio higher than 1 are bought more often by beer buyers. Reproduced from Johansen D, Friis K, Skovenborg E, Grønbaek M. Food buying habits of people who buy wine or beer: cross sectional study. *BMJ*. 2006;332(7540):519–522. Copyright 2006, with permission from BMJ Publishing Group Limited.

accrued from drinking wine have not been unequivocally separated from the wine drinkers' generally healthier diet.

Reverse Causality

It seems patently obvious that for an exposure to a drug to cause a disease, use of the drug must precede the onset of disease. Determining this with certainty is one of the criteria for establishing causality. But the temporal sequence is not always that clear-cut. We saw an example of this problem when discussing the study purportedly showing that coffee drinking increased the risk of pancreatic cancer. Here the symptoms of GI disease in the control group had resulted in them consuming less coffee. This phenomenon is called "reverse causality." In 1953, Jeremy Morris published in the *Lancet* one of the most influential papers ever written in establishing the benefit of exercise for reducing the risk of heart attack. In it he compared the rate of heart attack in London bus drivers, who sat almost all day, with bus conductors, who had to run up and down the stairs (these were the famous red double-decker buses) collecting tickets. The rate of heart attack in the drivers was about double that for the conductors and suggested a strong protective effect of exercise. But what if the job selection had been influenced by preexisting risk factors? Did men with high blood pressure and who were already at greater risk for heart attack become drivers, or had their doctors told them not to become a conductor because of poor health? This would be an example of reverse causality; but in this study Morris and his colleagues were able to rule out this type of bias by checking the health status of the workers before they started working. Additional studies of other active workers like postmen (mailmen), who in much of England walk their route, found they had lower rates of heart attack than sedentary male telephone operators, confirming the important role of exercise.[14]

Reverse causality occurs when the time sequence of the exposure disease association is reversed. Reverse causality may occur in studies examining whether people with "positive aging stereotypes" (people who perceive older age as having personal and social benefit) actually survive longer in older age than individuals who view aging more negatively. There is a good deal of research to support this hypothesis, but much of it inadequately controls for temporality. Respondents are often asked these questions in middle age (some are even asked in old age), and the concern is that those who are unhealthy and at higher risk of dying as a result of their illness may also hold more negative aging stereotypes. Even studies designed to exclude physically ill subjects cannot guarantee they are excluding people with early stages of disease, who have not been diagnosed with any particular condition but simply feel lousy, don't want to be answering research questions, and respond accordingly. This bias will always produce what appears to be a positive association between negative age stereotyping and earlier death.

My colleagues and I have been studying whether the use of antibiotics early in life increases the risk of childhood asthma. This interest is driven by the "hygiene hypothesis," which postulates that children who are exposed to bacteria soon after being born develop a much more robust immune system that protects them against asthma and other allergic diseases. Antibiotics would reduce the exposure to bacteria and may possibly suppress the immune response. The difficulty in studying this problem lies in the use of antibiotics to treat early wheeze and other symptoms of developing, but not yet diagnosed, asthma. In this case, an association between antibiotics and asthma may simply reflect the drugs being used to treat early asthma rather than being a cause of it. This special type of reverse causality, with early symptoms of the disease leading to an increased use of the same drug being studied as a risk factor for the disease, is called "protopathic" (or early disease) bias. We designed our study to limit the early antibiotic exposure to the first six months of life and the asthma diagnosis to being no earlier than three years of age to try and separate the exposure from the start of disease. We observed a modest increased risk of asthma in the antibiotic-exposed children, but the uncertainties in diagnosing asthma make it possible that protopathic bias still influenced the observed association.[15]

Choice of Comparator

I commented in an earlier chapter that risk always involves a comparison, and one of the most difficult decisions facing a researcher is what comparison group should be used when assessing the risk of disease. In study-ing whether exposure to a drug causes a bad outcome, we assume that the individuals taking the drug are comparable to those not taking it (the con-trols). The choice of inappropriate controls can lead to incorrect conclu-sions about a drug's effects. One of the most important assumptions is that the individuals not taking the drug are equally as sick as those using it. In practice, non-medicated ill patients are likely to have a different and usually milder form of illness than are medicated patients. Associations between the drug and subsequent harmful effects cannot be easily disentangled from differences due to the severity of illness.

For example, if we are studying whether a drug used to treat pregnant women with epilepsy increases the risk of birth defects in their children, what control group should be used? Women with epilepsy but not being treated with a drug may be considered, but they are likely to have a less severe form of epilepsy. This is important if epilepsy is itself a risk factor for birth defects (indication bias, discussed above). Similarly, if the epilepsy is treated with another type of drug, these patients may be considered as a control group, but here also the doctors treating these patients may decide which drug to prescribe based on nuanced differences in the presenting symptoms. These decisions themselves may reflect important variation in the disease which jeopardizes the validity of the association being studied.

Consider how many choices there are in selecting to whom smokers should be compared in a study to see if smoking increases the risk for dis-ease. First, we could calculate the number of cigarettes smoked per day, per week, or per year. Then we could form groups based on the number of daily cigarettes, which could result in two, three, four, five or more groups (1–5, 6–10, 11–15, and so on). The comparison could be the lowest dichot-omy, lowest tertile, lowest quartile, or quintile. Or the investigator could use some arbitrary low figure, say 100 or fewer cigarettes per year, or use no cigarettes smoked ever. Perhaps a more lenient referent of no cigarettes in the last five (pick a number) years is selected, or no cigarettes and no form of tobacco from pipes or anything else. All of these strategies have been used in smoking studies to select a control group. What is worrying is that the choice of comparator can influence study results, with positive results being found with one comparator but not another. Even more worrying is that the choice of comparator may be made during the statistical analysis and selected to emphasize statistical significance. Research reports rarely say why or when the comparator was selected, and the reader of a research report often cannot tell if a pre-specified hypothesis has been tested, or whether a new hypothesis is being created. As we will discuss in the chapter on pooling data, this matters a great deal in how research findings should be interpreted. Cigarette smoking is undoubtedly a health risk and is used here only as one example of how choice of comparator can bias research results, but this bias leads to false conclusions about many common diseases.

Lumping or Splitting Disease Diagnoses

It would be unsatisfying to have a clinician who treated her patient's condition using a broad rubric of disease, such as "cancer," "heart disease," or "respiratory illness." Your doctor's failure to define the specific type of breast or brain tumor would be alarming, but some researchers do this not infrequently. Researchers often group congenital malformations within a single organ system, such as the heart. This infers that risks identified with one type of cardiovascular malformation have evidentiary value with respect to another type of cardiac malformation. This assumption is completely unwarranted. Writing in 1984 on the problems in classifying congenital malformations, I suggested that "very little can be learned from studies grouping all malformations together. Thus analysis of specific defects or natural groupings of them based on their embryological development becomes necessary." And "only detailed examination of each individual case is likely to differentiate the specific etiology."[16]

It seems obvious that one would not lump cancer and heart disease together, but lumping can pose a more subtle problem. Suppose all malformations of a specific organ such as the heart might be safely lumped. Indeed, early studies of cardiovascular malformations often did lump them into a single category. The reason for this was largely to improve the statistical power of studies to detect significant associations. However, this ignored the biological, anatomical, and developmental heterogeneity in cardiac defects and precluded any sensible interpretation of the results. The classification of cardiac malformations has evolved along with increasing knowledge of the heart's embryological development and, in recent times, the influence of genetic polymorphisms.

In 2007 Botto and colleagues considered embryological development in 4,703 heart abnormality cases in the United States National Birth Defects Prevention Study to provide the most accurate method of classifying cardiovascular malformations. Their classification scheme consisted of 12 major groups of cardiac defect and 86 subcategories based on cardiac phenotype, complexity, and extra-cardiac anomalies. They also emphasize the tentative nature of classifying specific cardiac malformations, even into meaningful groups based on embryological development: "At the current state of knowledge, such pooling should be done with caution, and findings by such large aggregates are best presented in conjunction with those by the main groups. For example, studies on conotruncal anomalies [a major group] are likely to be more informative if they present also findings on the main groups (e.g. tetralogy of Fallot, truncus arteriosus, and so on) rather than a single risk estimate for conotruncal anomalies. One reason is that empiric evidence for or against a common pathogenesis or set of risk factors for these large aggregates is limited."[17]

Correlation Is Not Causation

One of the leading sources of public confusion about disease causation is the apparent linkage in time between the increased prevalence of disease and the appearance of a new potential harmful exposure. Autism is often diagnosed at the same time a child's vaccinations are given; ipso facto the two are connected. Add some publicized poor science from the laboratory and plaintiff's lawyers hungry for class action suits to the mix, and in much of the public's mind the causal link is considered confirmed. Epidemiologists call these unrelated links in time and space "ecological correlations," and life is full of them. Consider the rapid changes to our lifestyles, different trends in what we eat, and our ever more sophisticated electronic appliances, and it is not surprising that changes in the prevalence of disease can be linked to increases in many exposures. Additionally, many disease definitions are constantly being changed and refined as knowledge about them advances.

The names of some diseases disappear: female hysteria is, fortunately, long gone, and late paraphrenia is now often called late onset schizophrenia. New nomenclature is created through combining earlier classifications: for example, autism spectrum disorder (ASD) combines several previously distinct classified conditions. Changing the definition of a disease makes it very difficult to track real changes in the incidence of the condition and creates opportunities for ecological correlation.

In medieval Holland the number of storks on the roof of a house was highly correlated with the number of children in the house, and in modern Saxony the number of home births rose as the stork population also increased. How are these correlations explained unless the old stories are to be believed? In medieval times the larger houses, with more chimneys, attracted the nesting storks; the larger houses belonged to wealthier families with children who were more likely to survive. In modern Germany, it is simply a coincidence that an increasing trend in births delivered at home occurred at the same time that stork populations were increasing. Box 6.4 demonstrates how statistical analysis of ecological data provides a veneer of scientific legitimacy over what are essentially meaningless correlations.[18]

Ben Goldacre, the irrepressible *Guardian* columnist who writes on "Bad Science," provided a recent example of an ecological correlation.[19] British newspapers and the BBC both reported that the use of antidepressant drugs had risen dramatically as a result of the economic recession. Sales of SSRIs, the largest class of antidepressant, had risen by 43 percent from 2006 to 2010. However, they had risen by 36 percent in the five years before 2006, that is, before the recession. There is no evidence for a link between recession and depression when a larger data set is used. Goldacre also points out that relying on SSRI sales is a poor way of measuring depression as these drugs are also used for many other conditions, for example, anxiety. Moreover, other depressed patients are being switched from older types of antidepressant to SSRIs. But this was not the whole story as other surveys showed some patients were being treated for longer periods of time. Although this was not a particularly large number of patients, it was sufficient to substantially increase the number of SSRI prescriptions without any rise in the number of depressed patients.

Box 6.4. Home Births and the Stork.

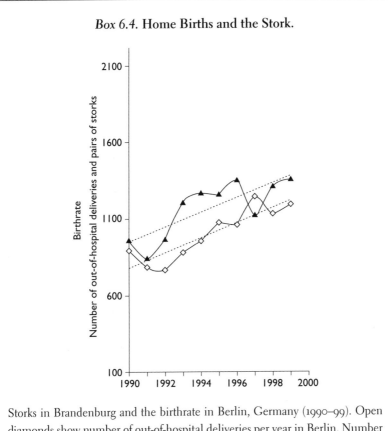

Storks in Brandenburg and the birthrate in Berlin, Germany (1990–99). Open diamonds show number of out-of-hospital deliveries per year in Berlin. Number of pairs of storks are shown as full triangles. Dotted lines represent linear regression trend (y = mx + b).*

*Reprinted from *Paediatric and Perinatal Epidemiology*, vol. 18, Höfer T, Przyrembel H, Verleger S, New evidence for the theory of the stork, 88-92, Copyright 2004, with permission from Blackwell Publishing Ltd., a Wiley Company.

In a series of studies conducted at the Hawthorne electrical company plant in Cicero, Illinois, from 1927 to 1932 industrial psychologists were examining the effect of the brightness of lights, changes in humidity, frequency of tea breaks, and other workplace conditions on worker productivity. To their surprise they observed that irrespective of whether the lights

Box 6.5. Very, Very Large Observational Studies.

It has become increasingly popular to create very large cohorts of research subjects who can be followed over time. Perhaps the largest study is the Million
Women Study in the United Kingdom, which involves more than 1 million
women aged 50 or older. This study was designed to look at the long-term effects
of hormone replacement therapy on breast disease but will also study a large
number of factors influencing older women's health. Another large study is the
Norwegian Mother and Child Cohort that is a long-term prospective cohort of
110,000 pregnant women and their children. This study examines a wide range
of environmental agents and their impact on pregnancy and the future health
of the child.

These studies are very valuable because they are able to obtain more precise
estimates of the risk from rare exposures with uncommon diseases. But many of
the biases discussed in this chapter apply regardless of study size. Indeed, one of
the anomalies of very large studies is that seemingly precise estimates of risk are
obtained, but they are biased (unlike very large RCTs). Also, large studies often
tend to examine multiple hypotheses and consequently may do a poor job investigating any single one. Very large studies have no advantage over smaller ones
in how much information can be obtained from individual respondents, in how
well it is remembered, or in how many known or unknown confounding factors
may be present. Journalists and the public often overestimate the importance
of very large observational studies, assuming that bias must have been avoided
when this is not at all the case. Smaller, more focused studies are often able to
collect more data relevant to one particular hypothesis and so test it with less
bias. It would be a mistake for national health agencies to focus more resources
into massive observational studies at the expense of more directed research.

were brightened or dimmed, or indeed whatever maneuver they introduced,
productivity appeared to improve. What the psychologists had observed is
that the very fact of being an experimental subject, irrespective of what is
actually being changed, is sufficient to induce behavior change. Despite
more recent suggestions that what is being observed is a "placebo effect"
or a "demand effect," in which subjects perform according to what they
think the experimenter's expectations are, the "Hawthorne effect" is now a
well-established phenomenon that is known to plague the correct interpre-

tation of research in all areas of behavioral science. If nurses, ambulance drivers, or doctors know their work is being evaluated, perhaps to assess the effect of some novel way of managing patients, this alone will likely lead to improvements in performance, irrespective of whether the behavior under study is having a real effect. Absent properly constructed experiments, the results of such studies can be highly misleading. It has been known for a long time that poorly designed educational experiments will suffer from the Hawthorne effect, whether they are the introduction of innovative teaching methods in the classroom (perhaps new strategies for teaching math) or studies of entire educational systems (such as building magnet schools). All will result in changes leading to temporary improvement in educational outcomes but many have no discernable long-term benefit.[20]

I ended the previous chapter with some critical comments about the overzealous nature of some ethical regulations governing clinical trial research, and we must now inquire whether clinical trials could be used to study harm. After all, if they are the gold standard for identifying causal relationships, why not use them to more conclusively identify harmful aspects of our environment? We have seen how difficult it is to confirm causality using observational methods.

Clinical trials randomize subjects to a therapy that, with some degree of plausibility based on prior research, is felt to be potentially beneficial. Although the principal reason for doing the clinical trial is to bring benefit, it can also tell us if the intervention has some harmful side effects. But if the principle reason for doing the trial is to see if a drug or chemical is harmful, this would conflict with the medical imperative "first, do no harm."

Goldberger could have tested his theory about the influence of diet on pellagra by randomizing prisoners to a superior versus usual diet to see if their risk of disease decreased rather than doing the opposite (chapter 1). This strategy would have provided equally compelling evidence that a deficiency in diet was causing the disease. There are no reports of long-term studies in the prisoners to see if the early signs of induced pellagra were ever reversed, which would have indicated some relief from the harm caused by the trial intervention. In Bradford Hill's trial of streptomycin for tuberculosis his patients surely could have been informed that they were entering a trial. Nowadays, patients would be told that if the experimental therapy (streptomycin) proved effective, those randomized to the control therapy would be first in line to receive it. We can be certain that there would have been no shortage of volunteers for Bradford Hill's project. But these trials were done in a different era, and we should not be too critical of them; modern ethical standards have undoubtedly led to some important protections for the subjects of medical research. Observational research, with all its attendant problems, remains our only tool for identifying the causes of harm from many medicines and from our environment and lifestyle.

SEVEN

Screening, Diagnosis, and Prognosis

If I move from Connecticut to California, the
average IQ of both places will improve.
— *Will Rogers*

Not too long ago, the American Cancer Society strongly recommended women practice breast self-examination and, if over age 40, have an annual mammography. For reasons that may seem obvious, early detection of a breast lump that may be cancerous allows more effective treatment and better chance of survival. Case closed? Screening for other conditions, prostate cancer, high blood pressure, high cholesterol, high glucose, and anemia, is now an integral part of modern medicine and health care. But is it that simple: is screening really effective? Are there risks of screening and any possible unintended consequences? Diagnostic and prognostic tests are commonly used in medicine, but how valuable are they? What do researchers who develop the tests — and the public that is advised to use them — need to consider to ensure that the public as a whole, and as individuals, are best served by them?

No test for screening, diagnosis, or prognosis is 100 percent accurate. They produce some positive test results in people who do not have the disease and some negative test results in those who do (respectively called "false positive" and "false negative" results). How can these tests be used in a practical way to optimize their effectiveness and to reduce the risk of them doing harm? Do the risks of falsely identifying a patient as having a condition during screening outweigh the chance of missing an early diagnosis? Is the risk of inappropriately treating a diagnosed but not ill patient outweighed by the risk of not treating some ill patients? Consider how an incorrect prognosis can lead to errors in how a patient is managed. These are all common dilemmas in the public health and medical arena and the subject of this chapter.

Screening is conducted in populations of presumptively healthy individuals to detect early signs and symptoms of disease that might otherwise be missed. Diagnostic studies are conducted where there is a suspicion of disease, either from screening or more commonly from patients themselves becoming aware of symptoms: a further test will confirm whether or not the disease is present. After a disease has been diagnosed, prognostic studies are done to determine the likely future course of the disease and how it should be managed. Each of these public health and clinical modalities relies on tests that have similar statistical characteristics but that also incur profound difficulties in interpretation.

Screening

Breast self-examination has been recommended for many years and is promoted as successful in the early detection of breast cancer. Most of us have read, or even know, of a woman who found a lump in her breast that proved to be a tumor that was successfully excised. The protocols for self-examination are detailed and clear: starting in her twenties, a woman examines herself monthly a few days after the menstrual period. Various strategies (circle, line, or wedge) are recommended for feeling the breast, and recommendations are provided for following up if there is a suspected problem.[1]

To examine whether breast self-examination actually reduced breast cancer deaths, a large cluster trial with over one-quarter of a million women employed in the textile industry was conducted in Shanghai.[2] The factories in which these women worked were randomly allocated to either the experimental instruction group (146,437 women in 260 factories) or the control group (142,955 women in 259 factories). The two groups were very similar at baseline on all important risk factors for breast cancer, including reproductive history and family history of breast disease. The women randomized to the instruction group were given very detailed instructions on breast self-examination (BSE) using techniques similar to the American College of Obstetricians and Gynecologists recommendations. They were tested for their BSE knowledge at subsequent time periods using silicone breast models, and their proficiency was reinforced by additional training at later time periods. For the next ten years the detection, treatment, and deaths in the two groups of women were followed and compared. The number of newly diagnosed breast cancer cases in each of the two groups was identical— 1.2 per thousand women—and the number of breast cancer deaths over the same time period was very similar—1 per thousand women.

Why did BSE have no apparent effect? Perhaps the women in the control group practiced BSE outside of the trial or had more mammography. But the study was able to show that the instructed women conducted BSE more frequently and in a more proficient manner than the controls, and mammography screening was unavailable to this Chinese population. The investigators were careful to follow up all the study subjects for a sufficiently long period and without knowledge of their study group, and it is unlikely these were sources of bias. Are Chinese breasts less amenable to BSE: do they have more fat, cartilage or other characteristics that make malignant tumors more difficult to detect? In fact the opposite seems more likely. It is reasonable to conclude, as do the investigators, that the reason for the essentially identical results in these study groups is that teaching BSE did not result in breast cancer being diagnosed at a sufficiently earlier enough stage of disease that therapy would influence the outcome.

Nonetheless, there were some important differences in the two groups of women in the Shanghai trial. Women in the BSE group were much more likely to detect benign breast lumps, which tended to be smaller than the lumps detected by women in the control group. Moreover, the number of benign lumps detected was greatest in the six months after BSE training. Regional lymph node involvement was the same in both groups. Despite rigorous training in BSE and more lump detection, this had no impact on disease diagnosis or mortality: there was no evidence that the diagnosis of disease was made any earlier because of BSE. Not only was BSE of no benefit, it burdened women with a false sense of alarm and the health care system with the unnecessary treatment of benign tumors. As currently practiced,

BSE cannot be recommended as a public health policy although it may be effective in some (undetermined) select group of women. Given current evidence, the onus is on those who propose such screening programs to document that it is effective. So far this has not happened.

Mammography screening, it is well established, reduces the risk of death from breast cancer in women aged 50 to 69 by about 15 percent based on the most reliable results from randomized trials. It is practiced by millions of women worldwide. For every 2,000 women screened over ten years, 1 woman will have her life saved but 10 women will be unnecessarily treated. More than 200 women will experience psychological distress due to false positive findings. This is not insignificant; it is estimated that almost half of all healthy women in the United States will have had a false positive after ten scans. The reduced risk does not differ for annual screening or three-year screening, and most programs now recommend a two-year interval between mammography examinations (in the United Kingdom it is three years). There is inadequate information to provide evidence-based guidance regarding the utility of screening women over age 69.

Whether screening in women aged 40 to 49 is effective is more controversial.[3] Certainly there are younger women who should be screened, particularly if there is a family history of breast cancer, which may indicate the presence of the BRCA1 and BRCA2 genetic mutations that carry an 80 percent risk of cancer. But even without these mutations, a family history of breast cancer is now thought to be sufficient to encourage younger women to undergo screening. If screening in younger women were shown to be beneficial, it would have to be more frequent than every two to three years as cancers that develop at a younger age are generally more aggressive and advance more rapidly.

In a trial in the United Kingdom with 160,921 women aged 39 to 41 who were followed for ten years, there was a 17 percent reduction in risk of death from breast cancer in those randomized to annual mammograms. In the group of women who actually complied with the screening guidelines there were 24 percent fewer deaths, but these results were based on a small group of women and could not be distinguished from a chance result. An important question is what was the rate of false positive results in these women that might have led to biopsies and unneeded surgery? Some 18 percent of the women screened experienced a false positive result over the course of the trial, and overall this was no different from that experienced by older women. This trial points to the importance of distinguishing clinical from statistical significance. If we were sure that screening reduced risk of breast cancer death by 17 percent in this age group, and if the false positive rates were acceptable, then the large number of women at risk would indicate that screening in this age group should be recommended as acceptable public health practice.[4] At present, uncertainty remains; the United Kingdom is currently moving toward extending screening to younger women and the United States toward decreasing screening in that group.

Prostate cancer screening and the usefulness of the most commonly used test, the prostate-specific antigen (PSA) test, is another controversial topic. The test has poor predictive value and a high false positive rate that can result in men who are not at risk undergoing radical prostatectomy with its attendant risk of erectile dysfunction and other significant effects on their quality of life. Six randomized trials of PSA screening that included 387,286 men have been conducted and, not unexpectedly, the test did find previously undetected cancers. However, for the most part these were not cancers that would have resulted in death as the overall screening effect on mortality from prostate cancer was not significantly different among the screened and unscreened men. A study in Finland estimated that 1 in 8 regularly screened men would experience a false positive PSA test and more than half of the men with one false positive test would have another false positive test on a later screen.[5]

In October 2011 the United States Preventive Services Task Force recommended that healthy men 50 years or older should no longer receive PSA screening. It was concluded that the test did not save enough lives to justify the far greater number of men who were made incontinent or impotent and suffered pain by being treated for cancers that would have remained indolent. It has long been recognized that many men die with a cancerous prostate—but not because of it. As happened when the same task force concluded that mammography in women under age 50 was not recommended, the PSA announcement was met with a firestorm of opposition. This came from both men believing, some no doubt correctly, that PSA tests had saved their lives by detecting early cancers and from urologists who, hopefully, were not influenced by the considerable addition to their incomes that flowed from PSA testing. Dire warnings that medicine was being sent back to the "dark ages" and that "thousands of needless deaths" would follow were made although no scientific evidence was presented to support these views.[6]

The task force took a more dispassionate perspective, basing its work on five randomized trials of PSA screening that included over half a million men and showed no improvement in death rates from prostate cancer ten years after screening started. The task force further documented that from 1986 to 2005 over 1 million men in the United States were treated for prostate cancer using prostatectomy, radiation, and hormone therapy as a result of a PSA test. Five thousand men died soon after surgery and up to 70,000 experienced major medical complications (20 to 30 percent of treated men suffer complications). Many proponents of screening cited a European trial as justifying PSA screening, but even in this trial 1,410 men needed to be screened to prevent 1 death and 48 additional cases of cancer needed to be treated, almost all of them unnecessarily. Other trials reported less optimistic results and in a large North American trial, screened patients were just as likely to die as those not screened.[7]

Why does so much uncertainty remain from these large screening trials even though the basic concepts for high-quality research (detailed in chapter 4) of randomization and long-term follow-up had been followed? First, the trials are designed to test population-based screening programs and as such they cannot be as tightly controlled as trials done in clinical settings. For example, in the men randomized to no screening there may be many who choose to be screened (52 percent in one trial), and in the men randomized to be screened some may choose not do so (15 percent in the same trial). In this trial, the difference in screening rates was fairly small (85 percent versus 52 percent), which may not be sufficient to show important but small differences in survival. Second, the screening level set for the PSA test will influence the study results. In some countries (and trials) the screening threshold for PSA is more than 2.5 ng/ml but in others more than 4.0. The lower threshold will always incur more false positive results and lead to more unnecessary surgery, but the higher rate may miss some aggressive tumors. Third, how frequently men are screened can range from annually to every four years. The shorter time period will detect more tumors that are unnecessarily treated, but the longer period may miss some rapidly growing cancers. Fourth, if the PSA test is accompanied by a digital rectal examination it may appear to detect more cancer. Fifth, how well positive tests are followed up and what the next level of treatment is will also influence results. For example, how many core biopsies are obtained in a diagnostic test? The more biopsies used, the less likely the discovered tumor is to be clinically significant. In one trial, 14 percent of men did not go for a biopsy after a positive test and among those that did, 76 percent had a false positive result. The success of therapy after screening will also depend on how patients with cancer are managed: by irradiation, hormone treatments, prostatectomy, or combinations of them, and these can vary considerably.

It is not surprising that those men who, as a result of PSA testing, have had a cancer detected that would likely have killed them are supportive of screening. Nor is it surprising that the surgeons who treated them might have the same opinion. However, these same surgeons must also be aware of the risks of harm from unnecessary surgery and treatment. What the task force did is compare the resources needed for population-based PSA screening of healthy men and the consequences of it. These are seemingly incompatible points of view, but no organized health care system can shirk the population-based perspective if expensive and limited resources are to be most effectively used. Nor should individual men be ignorant of the risks they face with this particular test. There is a much greater likelihood that they will be unnecessarily treated and suffer serious consequences than there is that a life-threatening cancer will be detected. Even the creator of the PSA test, Dr. Richard Ablin, has called its widespread use a "public health disaster." Given the scientific evidence currently available, even with

Box 7.1. Two Major Sources of Screening Bias.

Lead-time bias

Screened   "survival"   survival owed to screening

/ _____ Dx ----------------- Death>>>>>>>>>>

Not screened

/ _____ Dx --------- Death

Diagnosis in screened is brought forward in time→ Survival always appears longer in screened

Lead-time bias in screening occurs because earlier diagnosis made in a screened group always appears to lengthen the period between diagnosis and death. This is simply because the diagnosis has been made earlier than it otherwise would be. However, the course of the disease from the initial dysplastic events in the cell to eventual death may be unchanged. For screening to be successful, survival beyond the normal time course of the disease must be demonstrated.

Length-time bias

Slow growing disease

onset _____screen___Dx

Fast growing disease

onset _____Dx --------- (too late for screening)

Bias is to detect more slow growing disease by screening

Length-time bias results from the screening test preferentially detecting slow growing disease. Rapid and more aggressive disease may force a diagnosis to be made before a scheduled screening. This bias also appears to increase survival, which is not actually true. If a rapidly developing disease is to be detected, screening must be done at shorter time intervals, which is often impractical.

its limitations, it is incumbent on the promoters of the PSA test in healthy men to develop credible scientific evidence in support of their claim that the benefits outweigh its risks.

Sources of Screening Test Bias

All the studies discussed so far that examine the benefits and risks of screening are subject to bias. Lead-time and length-time bias, two classic screening trial problems, are shown in box 7.1. Other potential problems are rooted in the following: screening trials attract healthier volunteers than are found in the general population, which may appear to increase survival and lower the mortality risk estimates. However, persons already known to have a disease or known to be healthy must be excluded from screening as including them makes the test statistics look more accurate than they really are. To obtain generalizable results, screening test trials must be conducted in populations that are similar to ones where the screening will be used in general practice.

Diagnosis

Ovarian cancer is one of the most dreaded of all diseases. Although advances in treatment have improved the survival rates of 20 years ago, only a third of diagnosed women live 5 years or more. The chances of survival would be substantially enhanced if ovarian cancer could be diagnosed earlier. The symptoms that bring most women to medical attention—frequent urination, bloating, and lower abdominal pain—are nonspecific and occur frequently in women over age 50, the group among whom most ovarian cancers are found. An accurate diagnostic blood test is needed, and CA-125 is one biomarker that is considered to be able to diagnose ovarian cancer with reasonable accuracy. We will use it as an example to look at some of the difficulties in developing a useful diagnostic test.[8]

For more than 30 years CA-125 has been known, and it remains the most promising biomarker for ovarian cancer diagnosis. It is a glycoprotein found to be elevated in four out of five women with epithelial ovarian cancer, and continued suppression of CA-125 levels after chemotherapy is predictive of a lower risk of disease recurrence and improved survival. Nonetheless, the value of CA-125 to diagnose recurrent ovarian cancer remains uncertain, and data from a large randomized trial showed that intensive CA-125 surveillance did not improve survival. In one study, when the normal test level was doubled (and measured twice for confirmation) it predicted 99 percent of the women who experienced recurrent disease; however, 25 percent of the women who tested negative also went on to recurrence.

Although the test results might look encouraging, the benefits of earlier diagnosis and treatment of recurrent ovarian cancer in women who are clinically well but have rising CA-125 levels has not resulted in a clear demonstration of improved survival. This may reflect either "lead time" or "length time" bias, discussed above. It has also been noted that patient anxiety and depression may be raised in patients "living from one CA-125 test to the next."

Sometimes diagnostic tests are considered for screening healthy populations, and CA-125 has been considered for ovarian cancer screening. Unfortunately, the important test statistics change dramatically when the prevalence of the disease drops. In the study that produced the diagnostic statistics, the disease reoccurred in two-thirds of the study subjects. However, in the general population of postmenopausal women ovarian cancer occurs in about 4 per 10,000 women. This low prevalence has a dramatic effect in reducing the number of women who would be correctly identified as having the disease by a CA-125 test (although it would raise the proportion of women whose disease would be correctly ruled out, but this is not the point of population screening). A CA-125 screening test with a false positive rate of 1 percent would result in 100 healthy women being subject to the anxiety and risks from biopsy in order to detect 4 real cancer cases for every 10,000 women screened.

Sources of Diagnostic Test Bias

A new diagnostic test has to be compared to a "gold standard," which is typically the best current method for making the diagnosis. For CA-125, paraffin-embedded pathology sections were the comparison. The gold standard may in some cases have more of a pewter quality, being neither very precise nor based on high-quality evidence. This is especially true if the standard test is an older one, developed before the advent of more rigorous research methods. Nonetheless, such a comparison must be made, and to test the usefulness of a new diagnostic test, everyone in the study must receive both the old and the new test. Diagnosticians using one test should not know the results of the other, to avoid influencing their judgment. Both tests must be performed before any treatment is initiated so that the tests are assessing the same condition. All test "failures" (for example, the test was inconclusive) need to be taken into account (like the intention-to-treat principle in RCTs). As it is quite rare for diagnostic studies to meet all these criteria, the quality of many studies is often poor (for example, when compared to treatment studies).

Prognosis

Prognosis often uses pathological or clinical data, such as that from cancer staging (for example tumor thickness), the presence of cancer gene polymorphisms, biopsy data, and other biomarkers. These are typically ranked according to a range of values that indicate the severity of the prognosis. There is interest in identifying tissue markers that will help determine treatment programs, for example, whether cancer patients will require continued chemotherapy after surgery or some other kind of adjuvant therapy. Since the recurrence of many tumors is quite common, accurate prognosis is important for survival. Progress is being made, although this area of research is at an early stage.[9]

Sources of Prognostic-Test Bias

What are some of the problems that plague researchers trying to find useful prognostic markers? The individuals being studied must be at a uniform stage in the course of their disease, including whether they are newly diagnosed (incident) or long-standing (prevalent) cases. The latter will always demonstrate longer survival as they are already survivors from the earlier course of their disease. It is also important to note where the cases are re-cruited from: patients in primary care centers will likely have less advanced disease than patients recruited at tertiary care centers. In prognostic studies, the length of follow-up is important: if it is too short, there will be few deaths and late survival may be poorly estimated. Loss to follow-up may also be biased with the very healthy or sick being more difficult to follow, resulting in, respectively, under- or overestimating survival.

It is necessary to understand how a prognostic factor was identified in a study. Was it hypothesized before the study started, or did it come after multiple manipulations of the study data, which could mean it is a chance result? Has the prognostic factor been replicated in another set of patients? If it is a continuous measure such as blood pressure, cholesterol, or tumor thickness, how were the high- and low-risk groups defined? It is difficult to compare studies if different prognostic cutoff points have been used. This was exemplified in Will Rogers's comment about his IQ, and the phenom-enon has been graced with his name. If Will moves from Connecticut to California, he is suggesting that his IQ is below average for his home state but above average for where he is going, thereby improving the average IQ of both states. (Sorry California readers, I didn't make this up.)

Let us suppose that two groups are investigating the prognostic value of high blood pressure. A Yale study has two high blood pressure groups with systolic readings that range from 140 to 159 and 160 and above. A Harvard study uses groups with systolic pressure ranging from 140 to 169 and 170 or more. (Sorry Harvard readers, I did make this one up.) Which study will have a better prognosis in the two defined high blood pressure groups? It will, of course, be the Yale study because the average blood pressure is lower in both its "high" groups compared to Harvard's groups. This assumes that high blood pressure has the worst prognosis for a particular outcome, but the example can be readily flipped if low blood pressure has a worse prog-nosis. Of course, individual risks from blood pressure are no different in the Harvard or Yale patients, but the risks from the blood pressure groups are. The Will Rogers "phenomenon" (more properly called "stage migration bias"[10]) is also a problem whenever comparisons are made in screening and diagnostic studies that have used different cutoff points to define their risk criteria.

Moving the age for full Medicare benefits from 65 to 67 became a popular talking point in the 2011 US Republican presidential primaries. It seemed common sense that as longevity increased, Medicare enrollment could be postponed and cost savings achieved. The candidates would have been puzzled to learn that the average cost of health care for people below the new cutoff age of 67 would increase, but so would the average cost to the system for people receiving Medicare at age 67 and older. How could the average costs of health care in both groups increase? This is another example of stage migration bias. The average costs below the new cutoff age are increased because that group now includes people aged 65 and 66, who are the oldest members of their group and thus likely to have more health care needs, costing disproportionately more than anyone in the younger age groups. Adding them to the younger group raises the average health care costs and their privately funded insurance premiums before reaching the new higher Medicare cutoff. On the other hand, the 65- and 66-year-olds would be excluded from the now older Medicare group in which they previously were the youngest members, with health care costs that were on average lower than anyone else's in the older group. Excluding them forces the average cost of Medicare premiums and medical care to increase in the rest of the now (on average) older group receiving Medicare.

Excluding the 65- to 66-year-olds from Medicare would certainly save the plan money, and the (at least theoretical) cost of health care for *individuals* would remain unchanged whichever group they are in and whoever is paying for it. Nonetheless, because health insurance premiums are largely based on age and preexisting conditions, average costs would rise in both the pre-Medicare and the Medicare groups. It would have been great fun to ask the 2012 candidates for the presidential nomination to explain why raising the age for receiving Medicare benefits would increase the average cost of health care in both groups!

This has been a very brief examination of three very important research areas in health care: the evaluation of screening, diagnostic, and prognostic tests. When compared with the vast amount of research done assessing medical treatments, these three areas are often underexamined in a critical way. Like treatment studies, where the benefits of treatment must often be balanced against the risk of side effects, these procedures and tests are always in need of a judicial weighing of the pros and cons. If the threshold for a positive test, say for high blood pressure, is moved "up" (made more specific), it will increase the proportion of people *correctly* determined to have the disease but it will also increase the number of people who have the disease but are missed. As the test criteria are moved "down" (made more sensitive), the number of those correctly diagnosed falls but so does the number of people whose diagnosis is missed. This is the "yin and the yang" of all testing procedures. There are methods for optimally reducing these two competing sources of error but not for eliminating them altogether.[11] Where the positive test levels are placed is not only a medical or public health judgment but also a societal, economic, and cultural one. The costs to health care systems of additional testing when only a fraction of positive screening tests are subsequently found to be correct has to be weighed against the cost of delayed or missed diagnoses. The task of the researchers is to make these options as transparent and quantifiable as possible.

EIGHT

A Statistical Sojourn

If your experiment needs statistics, you ought
to have done a better experiment.
— *Ernest Rutherford*

If you do everything you should do, and do not do anything you
should not do, you will according to the best available statistics,
live exactly eighteen hours longer than you would otherwise.
— *Logan Clendening*

Causation is not demonstrated or proven by statistical analysis alone; the process for deciding causality is in part empirical, but it is also largely based on the strength of the methodology of the studies from which the data was derived. We have discussed how RCTs lead directly to causation conclusions. There is also an experiential element to recognizing causation; past experience informs us as to what types of preliminary evidence may, or are unlikely to, lead to a causation conclusion. If statistics gives you heartburn by all means skip this chapter, but I encourage you to give it a try; in addition to study methodology, which is discussed throughout the rest of this book, the second major element that is fundamental to understanding what conclusions can be drawn from a study lies in the quantitative results and in how numerical data should be interpreted.

The steps to determining causation start with the design of a valid study by using an appropriate and scientifically sound methodology, which is a largely nonstatistical exercise (the statistical part is deciding how large the study should be). The second stage is documenting how strong the association is between a risk factor and a disease (or a treatment and a cure) and determining how much of a role chance might have played in the collected data—this is where statistical methods largely come into play. Rutherford's comment about not needing statistics if the experiment is well designed is only partially correct. It is true, well-designed randomized trials often require minimal statistical analysis to answer the primary question; however, Rutherford was a physicist who benefited from generally reliable data. Biological and social data that are derived from observational epidemiology are much more variable and almost always in need of careful statistical analysis to tease out the experimental results. The third stage in documenting causality, one largely ignored until the last 20 years, depends on how the association observed in a study compares to the results of similar studies and to the entire body of research on the topic. It is very rare for a single study to be considered to have produced sufficient evidence to demonstrate a causal association.

What Is a Statistical Association?

What is an association in data analysis? It is the distribution of data points for two linked factors. In its simplest form this may be the correlation of two trend lines, for example, we saw previously that as the size of the stork population in Saxony increased, so did the number of home births. But correlation (another word for association) is not causation (sadly, these were unrelated trend lines and the stork hypothesis was not supported). Another common association is shown in figure 8.1, which presents the crucial pattern of data from a clinical trial. It might also represent the data from a prospective risk factor study, the only difference being that the allocation to treatment or control would be by usual choice or practice and not randomized. This 2 × 2 table is the fundamental architecture of data produced by prospective (or forward-looking) studies. There are equivalent 2 × 2 tables for retrospective designs and for screening and other studies (discussed below) and there are numerous other complex forms of presenting data, but the 2 × 2 table, embedded in all studies either transparently or not, almost always incorporates the key information produced by a medical study, and the most important statistics are the ones needed to interpret it.

Disease

	Yes	No	Total
Treated	a	b	$n1$
Control	c	d	$n0$

Rate in treated group = $a/n1$

Rate in control group = $c/n0$ Relative Risk (Risk Ratio) (RR) = $\dfrac{a/n1}{c/n0}$

Risk Difference (RD) = $a/n1 - c/n0$

Number Needed to Treat (NNT) for one person to benefit from therapy = $1/RD$

Odds Ratio (OR) = $\dfrac{ad}{bc}$

Figure 8.1. Structure of a study to Evaluate the Effect of Treatment

---

Box 8.1. The Effect of Baseline Risk on Number Needed to Treat.

Effect of baseline risk on NNT

- Baseline risk = 1%   RR = 0.75
  Risk with therapy = 0.75%
  RD = 1−0.75 = 0.25%
  NNT = 100/0.25 = 400

- Baseline risk = 10%   RR = 0.75
  Risk with therapy = 7.5%
  RD = 10−7.5 = 2.5%
  NNT = 100/2.5 = 40

Even though the relative risk is constant in populations with different baseline risk, the risk difference is greater in the high-risk population, and its derivative, the NNT, correspondingly smaller. In the high-risk population 40 patients need to be treated for the therapy to help 1 patient versus 400 in the low-risk population. This is one reason why the effects of a therapy, documented in clinical trials which are often conducted in high-risk populations, have a smaller effect when the therapy is made available to broader populations that usually include lower-risk patients.

Figure 8.1 shows the total number of patients who received the experimental intervention (n1) and the total number in the control group (n0), and among those receiving the intervention, the number (a) who had an event (for example, recovered, or did not recover, or died) and the number (b) who did not have the event. The same numbers are reported respectively for the control group (c, d). From these, can be calculated the risk of the event in the experimental and control groups (a/n1 and c/n0), and the relative risk (RR = a/n1 ÷ c/n0) and the risk difference (RD = a/n1 − c/n0). Another basic statistic, calculated from the RD, is the number needed to treat, which is simply (NNT = 1/RD). This is the number of patients who need to be treated with the therapy in order to have one success that can be owed to the therapy. If the study is assessing harm, the same statistic simply changes its label to NNH (number needed to harm).

Chance and Statistical Significance

If the risk of an event is the same in both the treated and control groups, then the relative risk is 1, which means there is no association between the treatment (or the exposure) and the eventual outcome. However, it is very unusual that the risk is exactly the same in the treated and control so that a RR of 1.0 is produced. We saw it in the study of breast cancer after induced abortion in 1.5 million Danish women and again in the breast self-examination screening trial of tens of thousands of Chinese women, but these are rare examples, and it is no coincidence that these studies involved large numbers of research subjects. Even in these examples, if the RR had been calculated out to more decimal places, it likely would not be exactly 1.000000.

We expect that, by chance, these risks will almost always differ from 1, even when there is no effect of the treatment or exposure. But how do we know if these differences from 1 are real and due to the exposure or treatment rather than being simply the result of chance? Does the size of the increased risk give us a clue? To a point, it does. Increased risks of over 10, if found in several studies, provide good evidence for causality, and this holds even if the studies are not particularly well designed. This is because it is very difficult to imagine a confounding variable that could induce a spurious association of this size. Moreover, it would have to be a confounding factor about which we had no suspicion or else it would likely have been considered in the research. Of course, a tenfold increase in risk is an arbitrary number, but this seems to be a reasonable rule of thumb. Most of the time, researchers are studying risks quite a bit smaller than 10, and so it must be asked at what point between no increased risk (RR = 1.0) and strongly increased risk, such as 10, can we rule out the play of chance? If the increased risk differs by a little, may we assume this is a chance difference, and if by a lot that it is real? It would seem as if some rules that are not arbitrary are needed for making this determination. This is where the concept of statistical significance comes into play.

To determine how much the observed number of events after an exposure differs from what is expected by chance, a Chi square ($\aleph^2$) statistic (O − E/E) is used to calculate the probability of the observed events (O) and compare them to a normal distribution against the expected number of events (E). If the probability of observing the number of subjects with disease who are also exposed to the risk factor is less than 5 percent, then the number of exposed subjects (whether too few or too many) compared to what was expected, is considered to be *not* due to chance. The association is said to be "statistically significant." How did this rule and nomenclature arise and is it as arbitrary as it seems?

Early in the nineteenth century the normal distribution (also known as the bell curve that shows the expected distribution or range of scores of an event, for example, the expected range of height or IQ scores in a population) was being quantified by the "probable error" (0.675 × standard deviation). The problem was to determine how extreme in the "tail" of the distribution a score had to be to no longer be considered part of the normal distribution. The notion that such an extreme value should be thought of as not due to chance and considered "statistically significant" was first introduced by Venn in 1866, and expanded in 1908 by W. S. Gosset (writing under the pen name, "student"), who proposed that anything outside 3 × the probable error (2.02 standard deviations) be considered statistically significant. The distribution tails +/−3 probable errors sum to 4.56 percent of the total distribution, which R. A. Fisher, in 1925, rounded to 5 percent. It is "convenient to take this point as a limit in judging whether a deviation is to be considered significant or not." Fisher (1935) later said, "It is useful and convenient for experimenters to take 5 per cent as a standard level of significance, in the sense they are prepared to ignore all results which fail to reach this standard." Fisher had started the significance/nonsignificance controversy that continues to this day.[1] It is unfortunate that Fisher used the term "ignore all results" because that is not how the concept of statistical significance is used today; rather it prioritizes study results as to those that merit more attention than others in future work. The 5 percent rule plays a very useful role in this respect. It has been instrumental in the search for numerous causal associations, and there are no generally accepted causal associations that do not meet this criterion.

The earliest statistical theory considered testing as if examining a single association, but in most studies several associations are studied and in some genetic analyses a million may be examined (which are discussed in other chapters). Clearly, when so many associations are being considered, a correction needs to be made to preserve the 0.05 level of statistical significance. Many options have been developed, but the earliest and perhaps still most widely used was developed by a Signor Bonferroni who proposed simply dividing 0.05 by the number of associations being studied. If 500,000 associations are being examined in genetics, this translates into a p-value of 0.0000001.[2] Chapter 6 discusses the bias that can arise from multiple comparisons.

Statistical significance testing is used to test whether the "null hypothesis," that is, that any differences seen between risk in the treated and control groups are solely due to chance, can be rejected (that is, the differences are not due to chance). If the probability of observing the different risks is < 5 percent then, according to tradition, the null hypothesis is rejected and a statistically significant difference is declared. Let us leave aside for now whether the difference is *clinically* meaningful. Importantly, failure to reject the null does not *prove* the null: the null (no increased risk after exposure) is not provable in a formal way. Absence of evidence that the risks truly differ is not evidence that they do not differ. It is commonly stated, "Absence of evidence is not evidence of absence."[3] Indeed, if the p-value is high (nominally $> = 0.05$), neither the null nor the alternative hypothesis has been disproved and a final judgment is suspended pending more research.

Importantly, significance testing refers to statistical hypotheses, not scientific hypotheses. Documenting an association as being robust (or even statistically significant) is by itself insufficient to support a scientific hypothesis. In epidemiology, that needs criteria like the Bradford-Hill formulation for causality described in chapter 15. R. C. Bolles put it: "One of the chief differences between the hypotheses of the statistician and those of the scientist is that when the statistician has rejected the null hypothesis, his job is virtually finished. The scientist, however, has only just begun his task."[4]

A question of great concern to scientists has been why does statistical significance testing quite often produce spurious results, or in the words of John Ioannidis, "Why are so many studies wrong?"[5] One problem is that most studies are designed to detect only borderline statistically significant effects. The calculation goes something like this: plan a study that can detect at least a threefold increased risk of disease using the usual p-value of 0.05 to rule out a chance positive effect and another p-value of 0.20 to rule out the chance of a false negative result. If the prevalence of disease is expected to be 15 percent, then 4,752 subjects are needed in the exposed group and the same number in the unexposed. Note that the sample size is calculated only to test the significance of the result at the edge of statistical significance. If the study finds a greater risk than anticipated, then the result will have greater statistical significance, but many problems with a research investigation discussed in this book can make that difficult to achieve. Some investigators may decide to set the p-values to a higher threshold when designing a study (1 percent and 90 percent instead of 5 percent and 80 percent), but this incurs studying a much larger sample (a total of 21,086 subjects in the example) with all the attendant costs, resources, and time that go with it, and many funding agencies will not provide the extra support needed to estimate risk with this level of extra certainty.

The difficulty with studies designed to minimally detect significant risks is that they have a reasonable chance of being wrong. Consider the accumulation of data in a study and what the 2×2 table would look like if it was calculated after, say, every five subjects had entered the study. We know the relative risks would be very unstable, they would likely switch from showing strong increases in risk to strong decreases, based on the small number of events in the early stages of data collection. Only when several hundred subjects had entered the study would the estimate tend to stabilize, and if the risk was as expected, only at the very end of the study would it achieve nominal statistical significance.[6] If the increased risk is greater than anticipated, the study will provide a more robust result than planned, but if the risk is lower it will not be demonstrated in the study because of insufficient study subjects (or too few study events, such as deaths). If studies were designed with more conservative estimates of risk, then more of them would produce replicable results.

The Fragility of Small Numbers

Many diseases and conditions occur at a rate of 1 to 2 per 1,000 and the unreliability of estimating risk for them is a major scientific dilemma. While not discussed here, analogous problems arise where potentially harmful exposures occur infrequently. Traditionally, rare diseases would be studied in case-control designs which solve the problems of disease rarity (see chapter 6), but concern over infrequent exposure remains, and increasingly studies of rare disease and uncommon exposures are being done in large databases or cohorts where other difficulties may apply.

The estimates of disease rates of, say, 2 per 1,000 are usually based on very large populations; perhaps the source estimate was 200 cases in a population of 100,000, and smaller studies are essentially a sample of some theoretical population. Any sample of 1,000 people is unlikely to have exactly 2 cases and may reasonably be expected to have none with the disease or possibly up to 10. Therefore, if one is conducting a study with 1,000 people exposed to a risk factor and a control group of 1,000 not exposed, imbalances in the number with disease are to be expected, just by chance. Let us suppose that one group has no cases and the other has four; if the exposed group happened to have the four cases the relative risk of disease is 9 (to calculate RR, it is necessary to add 0.5 to all the cells in the 2 × 2 table if one of them is a zero). Using statistical significance as a guide, it would take an imbalance of 0 and 7 in the two groups to reach statistical significance (RR = 15, p = 0.034), and imbalances this size and beyond would be deserving of further study. If the imbalance had favored the control group, a strong 93 percent reduced risk of exposure would be seen (RR = 0.07, p = 0.034).

Two observations follow from this simple example. First, given the play of chance in finding uneven distributions of rare disease between groups of exposed and unexposed subjects, it is useful to have some guideline, based on statistical significance, to delineate the point at which the imbalance may become more meaningful. Second, it is not infrequently said when reporting study results that if only a study were larger, then the risk estimate would become statistically significant. This, of course, assumes that the risk estimate would stay the same and we simply gain more confidence in it because of the larger study size. In fact, if the risk estimate is based on small numbers, it will almost certainly change with the addition of more study subjects, and, most likely, it will move towards the null, thereby demonstrating reduced or no increased risk. Importantly, this is also the tendency even if the relative risk had achieved nominal statistical significance. Risk estimates based on small numbers are not robust and are unlikely to be replicated in other studies. Statistical significance is not itself a guarantee that a real association between a risk factor and a disease has been observed. As we will discuss in chapter 13, replication of statistically significant results is a much more powerful indicator that an association is real.

It is useful to appreciate that studies that observe no cases of disease where some may have been expected still provide an estimate of risk. Finding zero cases is of some consequence even if the sample was small. If the risk of disease is 2 per 1,000 and only 250 people are studied, there was a 50 percent chance of seeing one case and not finding one does provide some, albeit imprecise, indication of risk.[7]

Why Are Many Studies Wrong?

Many meta-analyses of studies often show that the relative risks, even though they are not statistically significant, tend to cluster above 1 rather than below 1. This observation is, inappropriately, assumed by some epidemiologists, especially plaintiff expert witnesses in litigation, to imply that there really is increased risk, but the studies just didn't have the power to detect it. However, study results will always randomly produce just by chance relative risks that are more frequent above 1 because the range of theoretical risk is so much greater above 1, ranging from 1 to infinity. Below 1 the range is limited, only going from 1 to 0.

Another reason why so many studies may be "wrong" stems from how significance is tested. Suppose a coin is tossed 1,000 times and tails comes up 525 times. Traditional significance testing would say this pointed to a weighted coin; the probability of tails coming up more often than heads in that ratio is smaller than 5 percent. But 5 percent is actually the probability of the coin coming up heads 525 times and any number more than 525. It has been argued that the preferred approach to significance testing is to compare what the probability is for the observed 525 tails if the coin was fair, to the probability of seeing 525 tails if the coin was weighted, rather than making a comparison to the null, which in this example is 500 tails. This is known as a Bayesian approach to probability and has been discussed extensively in the literature but has not supplanted traditional methods of significance testing.[8] The statistician Leonard Savage has demonstrated that classical statistical methods overestimate the number of significant results by a factor of 10 compared with a Bayesian approach. This may be a contributing factor as to why so many studies produce statistically significant results that do not stand the test of replication. Interestingly, as we will see later in this chapter, the statistical estimation of the benefits and risks of screening procedures does use a Bayesian strategy that includes something called pretest probabilities.

It has been suggested that the 5 percent level of significance is an arbitrary criterion, but, as discussed above, it is hard to support this notion as it has been enshrined in the statistical and research literature for over a century, has a solid statistical rationale, and has found widespread acceptance. Many widely used scientific tests and standards have equally well-established normal values (IQ = 100) and decision points (such as, hypertension 160/100; obesity > 30 kg/m2; high LDL cholesterol 160–189; hyperglycemia > 10 mmol/l).

All of the statistics calculated from the 2 × 2 table should be presented with their 95 percent confidence intervals (CI), although in the secondary reports of research, such as in the media, these are often ignored. The 95 percent confidence interval is interpreted as representing the range of estimates that the calculated estimate would fall within 95 times if the experiment were to be repeated 100 times. The usual presentation looks like this: RR = 3.6 95%CI 3.0–4.8 (as noted, the interval is not symmetrical because on the lower side it is limited by zero but on the upper by infinity). In some circumstances, 90 percent or 99 percent confidence intervals are calculated, by tradition, but never 94 percent or 96 percent. It is now widely agreed that investigators should report actual descriptions of data (for example, risk estimates with confidence intervals) or exact probability values (for example $p = 0.023$) and not simply make reference to standardized values (for example $p < 0.05$).

The confidence interval also tells us something about statistical significance. If the 95 percent CI includes 1, then the p-value is more than 0.05 and the estimate does not meet nominal statistical significance. If it excludes 1, nominal significance is met. For example, a relative risk of 2.0 95%CI 1.2–3.0 is statistically significant and is interpreted as there being 95 percent confidence that the increased risk (RR − 1) lies between 20 percent and 200 percent. If the decreased risk is 0.5 95%CI 0.8–0.2, the reduced risk (1 − RR) lies with 95 percent confidence between 20 percent and 80 percent. How close the confidence interval is to 1 estimates how robust the result is. For example, if it is 1.1 on the lower bound of a positive risk, or 0.9 on the upper bound for a reduced risk, the result is of borderline statistical significance and cannot be considered a strong result. The result may be due to chance, even though in this particular study it meets the criteria for nominal significance. A great many results in epidemiology are of this type, largely because the study sizes were designed to be the smallest possible to obtain a significant result.

Despite some movement away from formal statistical testing in the epidemiological literature, it is still widely used in most clinical research, in genetics, and in regulatory proceedings. The legal environment highlights the difficulty; here a judgment must be rendered. Whereas a researcher can do another experiment or look for replication by others, a judicial decision cannot be delayed for further research. Nor can a clinician postpone treatment while waiting for further research, which may explain why statistical testing has persisted in legal proceedings and in the clinical literature. Modern geneticists are studying hundreds of thousands of statistical associations (see chapter 10) and must use the filter of significance testing to help them prioritize the associations of primary interest. Regulatory agencies, like the FDA, require firm guidelines for assessing the safety of drugs, and it is important that their decisions do not appear ad hoc, and so for them significance testing continues to play an important role in decision making. In epidemiology, no causal association has been documented that did not also meet the traditional criteria for statistical significance.

Data from Retrospective Studies

To this point we have discussed the 2 × 2 tables from a prospective study or from a clinical trial, but what does an association from a retrospective study look like? They are remarkably similar. If in figure 8.1 we replaced treated and control with diseased (or case) and not diseased (control), and event or no event with exposed and not exposed to a risk factor, we have the basic table for a retrospective study. The structure of this table reflects the architecture of the essential data from a retrospective study, typically called a "case-control study," which starts with the assembly of the cases, subjects with a disease and those without the disease, the controls. The case-control study investigates whether the *exposure* to a risk factor of interest differs between the cases and the controls. For example, do cases of the brain tumor glioblastoma have greater exposure to cell phones than a control group of healthy patients? All of the caveats discussed earlier about the need to distinguish a real association from one occurring by chance apply with equal force here.

Because the cases in a retrospective study are often collected without reference to the population from which they arise—the cases are simply collected as an opportunistic sample—this research design does not permit the calculation of disease risk in an exposed population compared to an unexposed one. The relative risk is not calculable. However, it was recognized in the 1950s, by Jerome Cornfield, that another statistic could be calculated that would in most circumstances estimate the relative risk quite well: this is the odds ratio (OR). If we return to figure 8.1, now relabeled for a retrospective design, OR = ad/bc. The circumstances when OR does not estimate risk are important: when the prevalence of the disease is more than about 10 percent, the OR will begin to deviate substantially from the RR, and when the prevalence is around 50 percent it deviates hugely. Fortunately, the case-control methodology is used precisely when the disease being studied is rare because prospective studies would need to be impractically large. In these circumstances the OR is very useful because it reasonably estimates the relative risk. Not infrequently, however, prospective studies and clinical trials, with quite common outcomes, will report their results as odds ratios, and these will always overestimate the true risk, whether the risk is protective or increases harm.[9]

Regression to the Mean

It is not unusual in studies of health care to identify a group of hospitals that may appear to be performing very badly—perhaps they have unusually high mortality or high infection rates—and then to implement a program of remediation that seems to improve the situation. Before declaring victory and considering the job done, however, it is humbling to consider the role of regression to the mean in bringing about this success. It is possible to rank all hospitals on their mortality rates, and this will form a bell-shaped curve with those having the fewest deaths at one (usually the left) end, those with average death rates will form the central body of the bell, and the hospitals with most deaths and the focus of our concern will be at the other end. If mortality had been measured without any error, then this would represent the true picture but it hasn't; there is always some element of chance at play in whether a patient succumbs and in how the statistics are recorded. (There are other concerns here about how some hospitals are selected to treat higher risk patients, but we will put that aside in this example.) Even without any intervention, when reassessed in a subsequent year, because the initial errors in measurement are not repeated, we would expect the hospitals at the extreme ends of the bell curve to have moved (we say regressed) toward the mean death rate represented by the hospitals at the middle of the curve. Moreover, those with the most extreme outcomes would show most movement toward the middle. Now, if the extreme worst hospitals had been in an intervention program to improve their statistics (perhaps by increasing their autopsy rate or implementing special mortality conferences), how would we know how much of any observed improvement was due to our intervention program and how much to the phenomenon of regression to the mean? We wouldn't, unless hospitals at the extreme had been randomly assigned to being in an intervention program or to a control group (chapter 4). Unfortunately, in many program evaluations, this crucial step is never taken. Of course there is a complimentary result: if the very best hospitals were measured again they would show worsening mortality rates, but this is often ignored. Regression to the mean is ubiquitous in all situations where there is repeated measurement over time and when those measurements contain some error. Remeasured blood pressures, cholesterol levels, intelligence quotients, and disability scales are all prone to regression effects. Many educational and social evaluation programs, when only the very worst (or, infrequently, very best) programs are studied, are misled by the effects of regression to the mean.

Regression to the mean is not a causal phenomenon, it is simply the result of chance, but it can substantially interfere with understanding causal associations. Many public health programs can be victim to it. I write this in Oxfordshire, England, where the police have reinstated the use of traffic cameras having noted a climb in accidents at various "hot spots." The placement of the cameras in the first instance was in locations where the highest rate of traffic fatalities had been observed, and after the cameras were in place the fatality rates in those places did indeed decline. Of course, by picking the highest risk roads for the placement of cameras, regression effects would mean that subsequent rates would have to decline. This would happen if the police had installed, rather than speed cameras, a picture of the queen. Even later measurements would show a decrease in accidents (it is also a feature of regression to the mean that measurements close to the mean at first measurement move away from it at the subsequent measurement). No doubt there are genuinely dangerous areas on the highway that traffic cameras may make safer, but this cannot be documented without undertaking properly randomized studies. Simply remeasuring fatality rates after cameras have been installed is not enough.

The Influence of the Type of Reported Statistic

Does the choice of statistic used to present data in a research report determine how influential the report might be to people who must use the data? In a series of interesting experiments, Naylor and colleagues showed data from a randomized clinical trial, reported in different ways to a group of clinicians, and found that it did.[10] For example, the following shows the same data reported in three different ways:

Number Needed to Treat (NNT)	5.5
Reduction in Events (RD)	18%
Reduction in Risk of Events (RR)	27%

The clinicians were more likely to rank RD as having the strongest therapeutic effect and NNT the weakest. The type of statistic used to report study results does appear to impact on how seriously the results will be taken; if two drugs with equal efficacy were reported from two different trials using different statistics, one might be incorrectly preferred over the other.

Multiple Levels of Risk Factor and Disease

To this point we have discussed the data coming from studies of association as if they were always reported in a 2 × 2 table and this is not, of course, the case. Exposures are often graded on a scale that can be categorical— for example, never drank alcohol, 1–3 drinks a week, 4–6 drinks a week, one drink daily . . . and so on—or they are continuous measures, such as height or weight, and they have been put into categories. The disease outcome may also be assessed in categories reflecting the uncertainty of the diagnosis or the severity of symptoms (both exposure and disease may be more properly analyzed in their continuous modes by using regression statistics, but these methods are not considered further here). When the data are analyzed in their categorical form, a series of relative risks are calculated, often grounded using exposure/no disease as the referent point, to assess whether there is increased risk with different levels of exposure (or by certainty or by severity of disease). These can contribute to a causality analysis, an important component of which is the expectation that as the intensity of an exposure increases, so should the risk of disease. There are statistical (trend) tests for deciding whether an apparent dose response is likely real or due to chance.

Screening and Diagnostic Test Statistics

The standard format for analyzing the data from a screening test is shown in figure 8.2. Here the data, coming from the Chinese breast self-examination screening trial from Thomas et al., discussed in chapter 7, have been calculated.[11] First, the likelihood ratio is calculated[12] and then the pretest prob-

	Cancer (Invasive + In situ)		
	+	–	Total
Self exam	864	132115	132979
Control	896	132189	133085
Total	1760	264304	266064

Likelihood Ratio = 0.98
Pretest probability = 0.007 (896/133085)
Pretest odds = .007/1–.007 = 0.007
Posttest odds = 0.007 × 0.98 = 0.007
Posttest probability = 0.007/1.007 = 0.007

Source: Data from Thomas, 2002: Thomas DB, Gao DL, Ray RM, et al. Randomized trial of breast self-examination in Shanghai: final results. *J Natl Cancer Inst.* 2002;94(19):1445–1457.

Figure 8.2. Breast Self-Examination Screening.

ability of a cancer occurring based on the experience in the control group. Next, the pretest odds is calculated, then the posttest odds, and from this the posttest probability. The gain from screening is simply the posttest probability minus the pretest probability. In this example, the pre- and posttest probabilities are identical (7 breast cancers per 1,000 women), showing absolutely no benefit from breast self-examination screening. Sensitivity and specificity are not calculated in this example because the Likelihood Ratio is so low. However, their calculation is straightforward: sensitivity = number of true positives/total tested positive; specificity = number of true negatives/total tested negative.

Finally, consider the PSA (prostate specific antigen) screening test for prostate cancer: levels in the range of 4 to 10 are considered intermediate and those over 10 are high. The more difficult clinical decisions concern managing patients testing in the intermediate range and the screening test statistics show why this is so. In one study, the pretest probability of cancer was 4.8 percent and the posttest probability for a PSA test result of 4–10 was 14 percent, a net gain of 9.2 percent from screening. This is an unimpressive result, but to understand it further we can calculate two additional test statistics: sensitivity = 0.67 and specificity = 0.80. This tells us that almost one-third of men who screen positive for prostate cancer will actually not have it, and 20 percent of men who do have cancer will be missed by screening. The principal difficulty with the large number of false positive results is that they often lead to invasive biopsy procedures and unnecessary treatments that can have significant negative effects on the quality of life for these men. Likewise, the false reassurance that one in five men receive is also of concern. Since many men fall into this PSA range, a test with better sensitivity and specificity is needed.

There are numerous excellent textbooks describing the statistical analysis of research data, and graduate students spend a very large amount of their time learning how to correctly analyze this data. However, as we have seen, formal statistical analysis is a relatively recent development in science. It is in trying to disentangle the uncertainties of observational research data that biostatistics particularly comes to the fore and can play a decisive role in improving the validity of the observed results.

NINE

Disease Clusters

The secret to long life is to keep breathing.
—Attributed to Claude Choules, the last surviving combat veteran
of World War I who died on May 5, 2011, aged 110

Some of my earliest memories are of sitting in the Morrison bomb shelter in our living room during air raids.[1] The shelter was designed to protect us so that we could be safely dug out should our house be hit by a bomb. I was born in Bradford, in the English county of Yorkshire, during World War II. The German Luftwaffe flew over us on its way to bomb more important targets in the west, particularly Manchester's industrial center and the Liverpool docks. When the Royal Air Force intercepted the Luftwaffe the Germans would think it more prudent to drop their bombs prematurely, turn tail, and retreat. Bradford was the victim of these offloaded bombs. Not being a target, the bombs fell in a random fashion over the city (our house was spared), but the pattern of shattered buildings often looked far from random: whole streets and blocks would be left intact but elsewhere half a dozen homes on one street would be in ruins. This is how randomness appears; it is haphazard, uneven, and the outward appearance is patchy not uniform. It never occurred to the dazed survivors to credit the clusters of bomb damage to some malevolent plan. Adolf Hitler and Hermann Göring, the Reich minister of aviation, weren't exactly popular, but none of my neighbors thought that the Germans had taken the trouble to target their specific house.

Cancer and other disease clusters appear in the same indiscriminate pattern. If several cases of a rare cancer appear in what seems to be a small locality, the search is on for a cause. Occasionally, as we shall see, it is possible to identify the cause of a disease cluster, but more commonly the cluster is almost certainly the result of the random and uneven distribution of disease spread across the population.

Many clusters, on closer examination, disappear because they have been artificially created based on spurious data. Some years ago there was a suspected cluster of miscarriages in the town of Groton, Connecticut. A doctor reported that he was seeing what appeared to be an unusually high number of his patients spontaneously aborting their pregnancies. Groton is also home to a major US Navy nuclear submarine base, and some of the patients were the wives of submariners. The obvious question that arose, not least in the press, was: were some miscarriages being influenced by the father's exposure to radiation? To answer this question, the investigating epidemiologist first had to determine if the cluster was real.

Miscarriage is not an easy condition to study because half of them go unrecognized. It is estimated that as many as one-third of pregnancies end in a miscarriage, but many of these occur soon after conception and before the woman is aware that she is pregnant. In all, some 15 percent of clinically recognized pregnancies terminate in a miscarriage. Early pregnancy miscarriage is not always easy to recognize as "spotting" or unusually heavy bleeding may result from either a menstrual period or a very early miscarriage. Many of these women do not know if they are pregnant, have never seen an obstetrician, and do not consult one about their unusual bleeding. However, women living in the town of Groton, or married to a submariner and aware of the newspaper reports of a miscarriage "epidemic," might be more inclined to visit a doctor to discuss their bleeding, and some of these bleeds, which would normally go undiagnosed, would be properly attributed to a miscarriage. A cluster of miscarriages would be born! Without proper investigation, it is obvious how this cluster might be linked to the exposure that had prompted the detection of an unusually large number of miscarriages in the first place.

To validate a cluster is far from straightforward. We must first define the cluster: is it the occurrence of disease within a census block, a city block, a town, a county, or some arbitrary circle drawn around a group of individuals with a disease (presumed to be associated with a specific environmental agent) and brought to the attention of the health department? There is no reason why disease patterns should follow political boundaries, and the latter strategy, by self-definition, is almost certain to demonstrate an elevated disease cluster. When considering an environmental exposure, say a toxic waste site, how broad a circle should be drawn around the dump? If it is too broad, or too narrow, the cluster will disappear. Indeed, is a circle the right shape for defining the cluster or do prevailing wind direction, stream configurations, or topography suggest another more relevant disposition? Disease clusters may also occur in time as well as space. A previous unremarkable rate of disease in an area may suddenly appear to increase. But how large should the increased rate of disease be and for how long should the increase be sustained for it to qualify as a cluster?

If we are studying childhood intelligence in Garrison Keillor's little town of Lake Wobegon, we already know none of the children will be below average! Clearly a stricter definition for lower than average is needed, but should this be a cluster of IQs in the lower quartile, the lower decile, or less than two standard deviations from the mean? There are no accepted criteria for defining a disease cluster in space, in time, or in the order of magnitude of the increased disease rate. Therefore, it's not surprising that most of the clusters brought to public attention are not validated by more rigorous research. The most common strategy for studying a cluster is to follow the disease rate over time, a period of "watchful waiting" to see if the disease rate declines to background levels (which it most often does). Many clusters are thought to occur around more permanent potential threats: Superfund sites, nuclear power stations, electricity transformers, and radio towers. When disease rates return to normal around these sites, absent any remediation, it is a sure sign that the initial disease cluster was likely a random occurrence.

Disease cluster investigation should be distinguished from industrial accidents, like the radiation leaks at the Three Mile Island and Chernobyl nuclear power stations or the Valdez and Gulf oil spills. They also differ from the natural disasters, such as the radiation leaks that occurred following the 2011 tsunami around Fukushima, Japan. These incidents define a geographical area or a special population that needs to be monitored for untoward health effects resulting from the exposure. Like the methyl isocyanate gas released from Union Carbide's plant in Bhopal, India, the health effects may be rapidly apparent, but in other cases, as at Times Beach, Missouri, with its dioxin exposure (discussed elsewhere in this book), they will not. In contrast to tracking the health effects of suspicious exposures, disease clusters are defined by an unexpected and usually unexplained rate of disease that demands investigation, first to see if it is a real increase and if so to locate the cause. To further explore the anatomy of disease clusters, it is instructive to examine some proven ones. The first example started with cat suicides.

The first sign of a problem in the small fishing village of Minamata in Kyushu, Japan, in the early 1950s was the strange behavior of the cats that occasionally fell into the sea and drowned. This "cat suicide," as the locals called it, began at the same time dead fish were noticed floating in the bay. Shortly after, humans started to exhibit disturbing symptoms themselves: slurring their speech, dropping chopsticks, trembling uncontrollably, and exhibiting other neurological symptoms that were often followed by paralysis, contorted bodies, and premature death. Initially, as it often is, infection was suspected (possibly syphilis or meningitis), but in 1956 epidemiologists identified very high levels of mercury in the local fish, in shellfish, and in patients.

In the 1930s, the Chisso Corporation, which had occupied a site on Minamata Bay for many years and which employed a large proportion of the village population who were not fishermen, began to manufacture acetaldehyde. The industrial process produced mercury that contaminated the bay in the form of organic methyl-mercury that entered the seafood chain. At that time in postwar Japan, the villagers' prime source of protein came from shellfish and fish, and eating the contaminated fish slowly poisoned the villagers who were unable to excrete the heavy metal mercury, which built up to toxic levels in their bodies. It is estimated that there were over 10,000 victims of this environmental disaster, which has many continuing legal, cultural, and social ramifications. For the student of disease clusters it had several important lessons.

The Minamata symptoms were highly unusual, mimicking in part some neurological conditions but also showing a unique constellation of other effects that were also very widespread in the exposed population. In most instances, the sick patients were readily diagnosed, and there was little doubt that an unusual and uncommon pattern of disease was being observed. The area covered by the disease, the cluster, was confined and quite well defined by local geography. Epidemiological research quickly identified a likely cause in the form of the exceedingly high organic mercury levels, and studies showed a higher prevalence of disease among the village residents who ate the most fish. In clusters like this where specific, definable conditions are met, it is generally only a matter of time and good epidemiological research before the culprit is found. But most often the disease cluster is of a relatively common and known disease, the increased rate of disease is quite modest, it is not sustained over time, and it cannot be linked to any unusual exposure. A researcher from the Centers for Disease Control once told me he had investigated over 100 leukemia clusters and not found a single one that was a sustained cluster over time or had any identifiable causal agent.[2]

Benoît Mandelbrot, a Yale professor of mathematics who is known for his discovery of fractals, illustrates the difficulty of defining a spatial disease cluster. Perhaps his most famous example concerned assessing the length of the shoreline of the British Isles, which is actually never completed: at every higher resolution by which the coastline is examined, every inlet and small promontory, or indeed every pebble or grain of sand, adds additional length. With increasingly finer detail, the length of the coast increases.

What level of definition is preferred for a disease cluster: the neighborhood, street, or house? Moreover, clusters are typically drawn as a circle, but this is by no means the obvious choice. Should they be ovoid or amoeba shaped? Is the wind direction a factor with more of the cluster being downwind of the suspected environmental agent? Should the presence of natural features, a forest, cliff, or highway be considered, and is altitude important? Cluster research, by definition, always starts with a retrospective examination of reported data. However, if the cluster is based on an existing pattern of disease cases, there are many possibilities for defining a cluster that will automatically force an apparent association with a suspected environmental agent. To complicate our problem further, clusters are not only spatial phenomena, they are also, as described earlier, defined by time. Deciding when the cluster began, what is defined as the first (or index) case, and when or whether the cluster has ended are also subject to uncertainty. Little wonder, then, that so many investigated clusters are never found to have a solution as to their cause, cannot be proven to be real clusters, and appear to reflect chance groupings of cases.

Many clusters appear to occur in the workplace. In Connecticut, the Pratt and Whitney Company (P&W) is a well-known maker of jet engines using a process that involves several chemicals that are suspected as being able to cause cancer. Around the year 2000, a group of P&W workers and their families at the North Haven plant noticed that several employees had died of the rare brain cancer, glioblastoma, particularly the type multiforme, which normally occurs at an incidence of about 3 per 100,000 persons. The family concerns were eventually heard by the company that proceeded to hire Gary Marsh, a noted occupational epidemiologist from the University of Pittsburgh, to conduct a study of the suspected cluster.[3]

Dr. Marsh and his team collected information about all the workers employed at all of P&W plants since 1952; this involved eight plants in many different locations across the United States. Not unexpectedly, many workers had retired or moved and many others had died. Fortunately, the company and the workers union had maintained employee records that helped considerably in the investigation. It was necessary to characterize the actual work done at P&W to determine what types of chemicals the workers were exposed to, the length of their exposure, and to investigate other environmental conditions. The workers' vital status had to be ascertained and, if deceased, their cause of death determined. This was a mammoth task, one of the largest studies of its kind ever conducted, but it was necessary to see if the initial reported cluster of brain cancers was confirmed.

Dr. Marsh and his team traced almost a quarter of a million workers and ascertained survival status for 99 percent of them; 68,701 deaths had occurred, and the cause of death was found for 95 percent. Surprisingly, when deaths from all central nervous system (CNS) diseases were calculated, the P&W employees had a 16 percent *lower* rate than expected and 13 percent *lower* for malignant CNS tumors (based on Connecticut statewide comparisons). Among workers at the North Haven plant, where the cluster was first suspected, there was an 11 percent increase in death from malignant CNS tumors, but this could not be distinguished from chance. There was also no association with duration of employment. When the occurrence of glioblastoma was specifically studied, there were 23 percent fewer cases for all P&W workers, and at the North Haven plant there was an 8 percent increase that could readily have been due to chance. Again, there was no increased risk with longer employment, and the subgroup of workers having the greatest risk were the salaried employees, who were least likely to have been exposed to chemicals.[4] This study continues, but it seems increasingly likely that the initial cancer cases formed an artifactual cluster. The brain cancer cases were, sadly, all too real but the cluster derived from a report that did not examine a sufficiently large number of exposed workers.

The science of cluster investigation has proved to be particularly difficult although it has engaged some of the best scientific minds from the beginnings of the science of epidemiology. Many cluster studies have involved childhood leukemia that, for several reasons, is particularly suited for cluster research. One principal question facing the cluster investigator is what to base the cluster on. When examining a potential cluster involving children's cancer, should it be birthplace, or where the child is living when diagnosed, or where a death occurs? The underlying question is the actual time the cancer started to develop, ideally when did the first metaplastic cell develop? For childhood leukemia, this is thought to be some three to six months before a diagnosis is usually made, in which case it would be plausible to base a cluster on where a child lived six months before the diagnosis. However, the time from diagnosis to death may vary, and children now, thankfully, live a very long time after their diagnosis, making place of death an unsuitable point for defining a cluster. Some cluster research uses multiple points in time before a diagnosis, but multiple comparisons (discussed in chapter 6) can result in difficulty interpreting the study results.[5]

Defining a cluster also depends on the hypothesis being considered for the cause of the disease. If an infectious agent is of interest, then studying school or nursery class clusters may be appropriate. It has been suggested that some leukemias are the result of a mutation in the father's germ cell, and testing this hypothesis in cluster research would involve placing the fathers of children with leukemia into some common historical spatial or temporal location, which is not an easy task. Investigating a putative environmental factor poses other difficulties. Toxic landfills, for the most part, are not being cleaned up and stay with us for decades. Studying potential clusters around them is made easier as we can track disease rates back in historical time and forward in real time. In contrast, we are limited when studying clusters that are (purportedly) quickly remedied. For example, diseases that may be associated with the 2010 British Petroleum oil spill in the Gulf of Mexico are best assessed with exposures relevant to the limited time when there was maximum exposure to the oil. Given a latency period of 20 years for some cancers, cancer clusters from the oil spill may not become evident until 2030, at which time measuring past exposures with any certainty will be very difficult.

In cluster research, as in any type of study associating an exposure with a disease, it does not necessarily mean that the disease in exposed individuals was necessarily caused by the environmental factor. Some individuals who develop the disease of interest within a cluster may do so for reasons unrelated to the exposure of interest. Clusters represent increased risk of disease, not certainty that all disease was caused by the exposure. We will see in a later chapter that, in legal terms, this is the difference between what is called general and individual causation.

A cluster can be considered to be a special type of association, one that links increased risk of disease across time and space. Even though a cluster may have been statistically documented to exist, it is subject to all of the association biases discussed in chapter 6. For example, there is a clustering of myocardial infarction on golf courses, which seemingly suggests that golf is one of the most dangerous of all sports. But of course, golf is not the culprit. Many men and women play golf at an age when they are most susceptible to heart attack; this is causing the cluster. When a cluster has been reliably identified, more studies, such as those for investigating harm, are needed to identify a plausible cause for the cluster. Sometimes cluster research can lead to unexpected major medical advances, and such a story is told next.

Time seems to have flowed by the small town of Lyme, just like the Connecticut River along whose eastern shore it lies. In the early nineteenth century, Lyme was largely known for being the summer home of the leading

American impressionists. Childe Hassam, Willard Metcalf, William Chadwick, and Allen Butler Talcott all lodged at Florence Griswold's house and created marvelous images of this tranquil area. That was about to change in 1975 when a group of mothers realized their children all had similar signs of rashes and swollen joints that were diagnosed as rheumatoid arthritis, an unusual condition in young children. Polly Murray, one of the mothers, first contacted the State Health Department, and David Snydman initially looked at the cluster before calling on a colleague, rheumatologist Allen Steere at Yale University. Steere, with a team of epidemiologists, infectious disease specialists, and rheumatologists, investigated the cluster in great detail. They considered various causes, such as infectious agents and air- or waterborne pathogens, but soon focused their attention on ticks. The children's symptoms began in summer with the tick season, and many reported being bitten by a tick that produced an expanding ringlike rash. The overall prevalence of children's "arthritis" was 4.3 per thousand residents, but among children living on four streets in Lyme the prevalence was 1 in 10. The first report of Lyme arthritis appeared in 1977 and described 51 cases, 39 of them children, whose illness was characterized by "recurrent attacks of asymmetric swelling and pain in a few large joints, especially the knee." The authors concluded their report: "'Lyme arthritis' is thought to be a previously unrecognized clinical entity, the epidemiology of which suggests transmission by an arthropod vector."[6]

Six months into their investigation, Steere and colleagues reported more details of the rash, now called "erythema chronicum migrans," and started to recognize longer-term neurological and myocardial complications. In a groundbreaking report, they identified the tick, *Ixodes scapularis*, as the likely source of transmission.[7] It wasn't until 1982 that Willy Burgdorfer, working at the Rocky Mountain Laboratories of the National Institutes of Health, discovered the actual bacterium transmitted by the tick. It was named in his honor: *Borrelia burgdorferi*. By this time it was recognized that the condition was not a type of arthritis, and the term "Lyme disease" came into common use.

Historical research shows that the first recorded case of what might have been Lyme disease came from Breslau, Germany, in 1883 and was reported by Alfred Buchwald. In 1909, a Swede, Arvid Afzelius, described the characteristic rash and postulated that it originated from *Ixodes scapularis*. In the 1920s and 1930s the link between the rash and subsequent neurologic, psychiatric, and other chronic conditions was being reported. But it wasn't until the careful analysis of the Lyme cluster by Steere and colleagues, and the work of Willy Burgdorfer in subsequently identifying the pathogen, that the complete natural history of Lyme disease and its consequences began to be fully understood. Lyme disease is now found in every state in the United States and in many other parts of the world. Understanding its causes has led to more effective prevention and treatment and to the realistic prospect of developing a safe and effective vaccine.[8]

TEN

Genetics and the Genome

They fuck you up, your mum and dad
They may not mean to, but they do
They fill you with the faults they had
And add some extra, just for you.
—*Philip Larkin*

Philip Larkin, considered one of Britain's greatest poets of the twentieth century, was right but not for the reasons he thought. It is increasingly recognized that many of the diseases that afflict us are of genetic origin, inherited from our "mum and dad." Alzheimer's disease, autism, cancer, hypertension, asthma, all have a strong genetic component to their cause. For some diseases, it has been known for many years that the condition was entirely owed to a genetic origin. Trisomy 21, also known as Down syndrome, is caused by an extra complete chromosome (number 21) that entirely explains the syndrome, although it can be manifest in a variety of forms. With almost daily regularity, the association of a variant gene with a disease is being reported in the medical literature and in the press. Research in this area began to be published at an almost exponential rate after the complete map of the human genome sequence was first described and published in 2001, and it has continued unabated. There is no doubt that genetic variation plays a major role in disease causation; indeed, it may play some part in the cause, or if not the direct cause then in the severity in expression, of all diseases. In order to understand how genetic variation influences susceptibility to disease, we first need to understand the structure of the genome.[1]

The Architecture of the Human Genome

The human genome, the name we give to the totality of our DNA, is made up of some 3.1 billion DNA base pairs, each base pair having two nucleotides, which are clustered into 22 autosomal, and two sex chromosomes, X and Y. Each person has two copies of each of these chromosomes, one inherited from each parent. The nucleotides along the maternal and paternal copies of the chromosomes are generally identical; however, the base pairs can occasionally differ in a population, and when this occurs we call the difference a polymorphism. If the polymorphic nucleotide is inside a gene it is called an allele, with each polymorphism having two alleles, one inherited from each parent. This is most dramatically exemplified by the X and Y sex chromosomes in which an XX individual is female, one X chromosome inherited from each parent. The XY individual is male, the X chromosome inherited from the mother and Y chromosome inherited from the father. The chromosomes contain approximately 22,000 genes, inside which the functional DNA resides, with each single gene containing from 500 to 2.5 million base pairs. The base pairs form the DNA that is famously in the shape of a double helix. The genome is something like the desert, with occasional gene oases interspersed in huge stretches of apparently barren DNA. The great majority (98 percent) of nucleotides (the desert) appear to have no function and so may play no role in disease causation; they include remnants of our ancestral past, not just as Homo sapiens but going back to our early evolutionary beginnings. The desert DNA contains bits of bacterial, viral, and parasite DNA, to which our ancestors were exposed, and it has become incorporated into the human genome. This has been called junk DNA. In fact, these huge stretches of DNA are being found to have surprising complexity, and some of it may be important in disease etiology; this research is ongoing. But it is most likely that the majority of this ancestral DNA is neutral with respect to disease susceptibility and does not increase disease risk. DNA variants that substantially increased our chance of disease would have been selected out of our genome generations ago.

That humans have so few genes was astonishing when it was first observed; rice, worms, and fruit flies have many more genes, and some scientists had predicted that humans might have as many as a million genes. It is now recognized that the combinatorial possibilities of genes and their interaction with each other actually create an extremely high number of possibilities for genetic variation and functional expression. Moreover, all but the smallest genes can be "spliced" in alternative ways to produce several different proteins, and it is proteins that form the animal's structure and produce or prevent disease. Even though it seems as if genetic discoveries are being announced every week, the role that many genes play in the function of our body is still not known; indeed, as the structure of the gene is scrutinized in greater detail, it is becoming less clear what actually defines a gene. Some genes have regulatory structures that are not even embedded in the gene that they regulate, and some genes are incorporated inside others (so much for "intelligent design"!). Almost half of the genome is made up of multiple copies of the same stretches of DNA, but these, as well as deleted stretches of DNA, can vary considerably among individuals. Their possible role in disease causation is discussed below.

The final major genomic structure we need to mention here is the haplotype. These are linked groups of alleles that always appear together and are found within and between genes. They are important structures that need to be taken into account in the search for genetic associations, and they may simplify that search by limiting the number of single nucleotide polymorphism (SNP) associations that need to be examined, but it is still unclear what role, if any, they play in human variation and disease susceptibility. In 2005 the first map was published that described the block structure of over 1 million SNPs across the genome. This and subsequent additions to the "HapMap" now guide the design and analysis of large-scale gene mapping studies.[2]

If proteins are the fundamental determinant of health and disease, how many are there? Genes are made up of one or more exons which are the coding regions for proteins. It is thought that as many as half of all genes have alternative splicing capabilities, each spliced section being an exon. Each exon can be mixed and matched with others to form different proteins from the same set of exons. However, some "proto-proteins" may also be produced that are again spliced into many different proteins. It has been estimated that the 22,000 genes may be responsible for making 2 million different proteins. Not every cell type contains every protein (collectively called the proteome), and these may be limited to a thousand different proteins being present in any one type of cell.

Large Genetic Variations and Disease Causation

The most extreme genomic variation is found when an entire chromosome is missing or duplicated. Fortunately, they are very rare, occurring in 1 to 2 per 1,000 births, which is not surprising because many of these are lethal and result in fetal death. The most common are: Down syndrome (extra chromosome 21), Patau (extra 13), and Edwards (extra 18); newborns with the last two syndromes usually die at birth. Turner syndrome (born as a girl but only one X chromosome) and Klinefelters syndrome (born as a boy but with an extra X) are the most common sex chromosome anomalies. Sometimes the tip of a chromosome is missing, as in Cri du chat syndrome, caused by a deletion at the tip of chromosome 5. For all these conditions, causality is well established, and since so many genes are affected, the syndromes are complex and disturb many organ systems and functions.

It has been known for centuries that some diseases run in families, and in their strongest manifestation, when parents are carriers for the disease (but do not actually have it), they will have a one-in-four chance that each child will develop what is called a recessive disease. These are diseases caused by a single gene variant and they are called Mendelian diseases, named after Gregor Mendel, the Czech monk who first demonstrated these types of inheritance patterns (although he worked with smooth and wrinkled peas, not people). About 1 percent of births are affected by one or another kind of Mendelian disorder although individually they occur between 1 per 10,000 and 1 per 100,000 births. Some examples are: cystic fibrosis, Tay-Sachs disease, and sickle-cell anemia. The genetic origin of these conditions was understood even before the actual gene responsible for them had been identified. Here, too, the causation of these conditions is unambiguous.

Gene Variation and Complex Disease Susceptibility

We now turn to the genetic origins of disease that are far more complicated. We call the diseases that they influence, complex diseases; they include cancer, asthma, and diabetes. In these diseases genetic variation affects a much smaller piece of the genome, sometimes a single nucleotide, but there may be many such small variants. Here we must introduce another piece of the genomic architecture: a single nucleotide polymorphism (SNP), which refers to a variation in one nucleotide among the genomes of individuals from the same species. The nucleotides are made up of four amino acids represented by the letters ACGT, and the string of letters in the same stretch of DNA among individuals is usually constant. A SNP occurs where the usual sequence is changed, for example, AACGTCG is changed to AACCTCG, a G having been transposed to a C at the fourth position. This change is a SNP: if the change occurs in one nucleotide, it is heterozygous, and it is homozygous if changed in both base pair nucleotides. A few SNPs within the gene can be sufficient to induce disease; for example, Huntington's disease is the result of three SNPs (the trinucleotide CAG) repeated 36 to 120 times in the *HTT* gene. Some Mendelian diseases also result from changes to a single SNP. On the other hand, a familial type of breast cancer is influenced by numerous genetic changes in two tumor suppressor genes, *BRCA1* and *BRCA2*, which confer a sufficiently large increased risk that women with these genetic variations quite properly ask themselves whether they should undergo a prophylactic removal of their breasts. But these examples are unusual. It is now apparent that single SNP or even multiple SNP variations in a single gene may increase the risk of disease by only a small amount.

The search for susceptibility SNPs has been greatly enhanced by technological developments that allow up to 1 million SNPs to be studied in genome-wide association studies (GWAS). These are a special kind of case-control study in which the DNA of a group of diseased cases is compared to the DNA of a group of controls, the actual DNA contrast being to compare the frequency of each of 1 million preselected SNPs between the two groups. In previous decades candidate genes based on research in animals or on theoretical considerations were studied. In contrast, the GWAS employs a hypothesis-free strategy: there is no prespecification as to which SNP will influence disease or whether it will increase or decrease risk. Clearly, with a million associations being studied many (actually 50,000) would meet the nominal level of statistical significance, and so sophisticated methods have been developed that correct for both the number of SNPs studied and the haplotype or linked structure of the genome.[3]

My Yale colleague Josephine Hoh conducted the first successful GWAS study, looking for genes associated with adult macular degeneration (AMD), a type of blindness generally afflicting people in middle age, and found one gene that explained a large proportion of cases with the dry form of the disease; another colleague, Andrew DeWan, discovered a gene for the wet form of AMD.[4] GWAS studies have now provided clues to the genetic causes of many other diseases, including Crohn's disease, types 1 and 2 diabetes, Parkinson's disease, prostate cancer, autism, obesity, coronary artery disease, bipolar disorder, rheumatoid arthritis, and asthma. Different responses to medications, such as antidepressants, also have genetic origins, and these have been studied using GWAS methodology. In March 2010, the National Institutes of Health reported that 779 areas of the genome had been implicated in 148 common diseases. The success of GWAS in identifying susceptibility genes is clear, but the clinical payoff that people have waited for—more effective therapies or screening tools—remains elusive. With few exceptions, the SNP associations have been quite small, many showing a less than 5 percent increased risk of disease, and so their utility as a screening tool is also limited. There are several companies trying to develop therapies, notably for AMD, but this is a long process and success is uncertain. It now seems apparent that the complex diseases are influenced by many SNP variants, each occurring quite infrequently and affecting several genes in concert, and so work is turning to looking at gene-gene interactions to see if this explains more of the risk for disease.

Sequencing: The Future Has Arrived

It is very presumptuous to write about the future in genetic research because whatever you describe, someone is probably already doing it: what the future really means is the adoption of new technologies into widespread practice. When the human genome map was largely finished, in 2001, it had taken several years and cost 2.7 billion dollars to sequence one genome (made up from several anonymous volunteers). By 2007 it cost 1 million dollars to sequence another, that of James Watson the co-discoverer of the structure of DNA. Whole genome sequencing is the term for mapping all 3 billion base pairs. Companies now advertise doing this for $2,000 and it takes a few days, still a formidable task if several thousand people required sequencing. The race to complete a fully sequenced genome for $1,000 appears to have been won by a US biotechnology company that announced in January 2012 that its Ion Proton sequencer could accomplish the task. But we have seen that the functional part of the genome, the oases in the genetic desert, take up only about 2 percent of the genome, and the genome that actually makes protein, the exome (the date palms in the oasis if this metaphor can be stretched any further), is a mere 1 percent of the genome. Exome sequencing needs to analyze only 3 million nucleotides. We have further noted that silicon chips with up to a million SNPs are already in use and the haplotype structure of the genome means that inferences to many more SNPs can be made, and so the gap between these research strategies is narrowing. Going forward, the major problem is more likely to be storing the vast amount of data produced by sequencing rather than the cost of sequencing itself.[5]

Exome sequencing and GWAS accomplish different goals. The SNPs found in GWAS are largely outside the exome; they are typically in the introns, the stretch of the genome within genes, dividing the exons, that does not produce proteins, and, as we have discussed, the identified SNPs may not be the actual ones causing disease. Because of the haplotype structure throughout the genome, and the selection of SNPs the manufacturers put on the gene chips used in GWAS, many of the identified SNPs are not in disease-causing genes, and the actual functional variants remain to be identified. In contrast, exome sequencing directly identifies SNPs and genes responsible for protein coding, and it is thought that 85 percent of all disease-causing mutations reside in the exome. This makes exome sequencing an efficient research strategy: studying 1 percent of the genome to find 85 percent of disease mutations.

Full exome sequencing has the advantage of not depending on SNPs that have been selected for the chips most widely used in GWAS studies — these are a mixture of randomly selected SNPs with a frequency of at least 5 percent across the genome and other SNPs especially selected because previous research has shown them to be of particular interest. These are called "tagging SNPs" because they identify a region of interest, but the identified SNP is itself unlikely to be the causal SNP; rather it is one that is in what is called "linkage disequilibrium" with it. The differences in the SNPs used in various chips confounds the cross comparison of study results, and current strategies of SNP discovery require that regions around the SNP, often the entire gene and flanking regions, need to be sequenced to find the causal SNP. Moreover, SNPs with a frequency of less than 5 percent are not included in the gene chips even though they may cause some rare disease or account for some instances of common diseases.

The first results from exome sequencing have been quite spectacular. Richard Lifton and colleagues at Yale University sequenced the exomes of a small number of children from the Middle East thought to have a rare condition called Bartter syndrome. But the sequencing identified a mutation that suggested a different diagnosis: congenital chloride diarrhea.[6] Other early exome studies are also using very small numbers of cases with extremely rare syndromes to identify the true causal mutations. Only when this is done, and an accurate diagnosis is made, can the biological pathways underpinning the disease be studied so that appropriate therapies may be developed.

Moving exome sequencing from the Mendelian diseases to the complex ones that are under the control of dozens of genetic variants is not a straightforward extrapolation, but the technical difficulties are being solved. In a recent study of metastatic melanoma, the most deadly form of skin cancer, DNA from the tumor (from 14 patients) and matching blood samples were both exome-sequenced and a tumor suppressor gene was identified with numerous mutations. These genes, when not mutated, act as a break on

Box 10.1. The Black Death and HIV/AIDS, Is There a Link?

Eyam in August 1685 was a peaceful village in Derbyshire, England, until a bundle of cloth arrived from London, destined for the tailor George Vicars. Sadly, it was full of infected fleas and George was the first to die of bubonic plague in an epidemic that over the next 14 months would claim the lives of 260 villagers. The plague killed tens of thousands in many villages and towns across England and Europe, but Eyam is remembered for the selflessness of the villagers, who took great pains to isolate themselves so that the disease would not spread. To this day, there are people living in Eyam who are descendants of the plague survivors.

Ever since AIDS was first described in the early 1980s it has been apparent that there were people who were clearly exposed to the disease; in those early days it was actively gay men who practiced unsafe sex, but some of them seemed immune from infection. Stephen O'Brien, and scientists from the National Cancer Institute in Washington, trying to discover if there was a genetic variant that might explain this protection, turned to the Eyam survivors and studied their DNA. They found in them a variant *CCR-5 Δ32* that occurred with unusually high frequency (14 percent). CCR-5 is a cell receptor that transports the HIV virus into the cell, but when the Δ32 mutation is homozygous, that is, inherited from both parents, HIV cannot infect the cell and these individuals are protected. Had the same mutation protected people against the plague? Other work suggested that the mutation in Europeans had become more frequent at the same time many plague epidemics struck, about 700 years ago, and the high prevalence of Δ32 seemed to match the European countries affected by the plague. Recent work suggests the story is more complicated. Areas with very low rates of Δ32, such as Asia, Africa and the Middle East, not only had early plague epidemics but the disease may have originated there. The plague spread from southern Europe to the north while the frequency of Δ32 tracks in the opposite direction. Nonetheless, Δ32 may have mutated in northern Europe and conferred protection in the later plague epidemics just as it does in the AIDS epidemic of the twentieth century.*

*It is conventional to write the gene in italics and the gene product in non-italics. For more detail on this current controversy, see Cohn SK Jr., Weaver LT. The Black Death and AIDS: CCR5-Δ32 in genetics and history. *QJM*. 2006;99(8):497–503.

uncontrolled cell proliferation.[7] In yet other work, ten children with undiagnosed mental retardation and their parents had exome sequencing that resulted in finding a different but likely causal mutation in each of six of the ten children; in all cases, these were new mutations that had not been inherited.[8]

Copy Number and Disease Causation

Copy number variation (CNV) was described earlier as being quite common across the genome, in the form of deleted segments of DNA or where a length of DNA has been replicated several times. By convention, a CNV is considered as being more than 1,000 base pairs long, but it is recognized that this misses, at least until the technology for studying them improves, what is likely to be an important number of shorter length CNVs. We now know that CNVs form an important component of human genetic variation and are a direct cause of many diseases and adverse conditions. CNVs are usually inherited although a significant number can arise from fresh mutations and may result in the episodic occurrences of rare or common diseases such as autism. Interestingly, the genomes of African populations have a massively greater number of CNVs than do any other human population, reflecting the much greater span of time in which Africa's hominoids evolved, the small size of the population that migrated out of Africa, and the even smaller number of migrants who were the progenitors of the world's current population.

CNVs can have a substantial effect on gene transcription and translation, the processes that produce proteins, so that the protein may not be made at all, or it may be made but in greater or lesser "doses" than normal. Inherited CNVs appear to be transmitted in a Mendelian fashion and account for most diseases presently known to be caused by CNVs. The GWAS technology designed to study SNPs has been modified to identify CNVs and is showing a remarkable degree of success even though it is only a few years old. One of the first reports showed strong associations of CNVs with schizophrenia, and subsequent work has linked them to a broad range of disorders, including attention deficit hyperactivity disorders, asthma, autism, Crohn's disease, developmental delay, diabetes, HIV, IQ, lupus, malaria, neuroblastoma, obesity, osteoporosis, psoriasis, and rheumatoid arthritis. CNVs have been found to influence tumor suppressor genes and so may have a role in the development of many cancers. At present, over 60 rare syndromes have also been linked to a CNV, and the evidence for them being responsible for a substantial burden of disease is growing.

The study designs for CNVs are in many respects not unlike that for SNPs, and the huge amount of methodological work done for SNP investigations can be carried over to CNVs, although some additional difficulties remain. One is the uncertainty of knowing just how a CNV is defined since some may overlap with others and the length may vary among individuals. These pose problems in statistical analysis and significance testing because the multiple comparison corrections remain uncertain. Nonetheless, these are not insurmountable issues, and it is likely that research in this area will be very productive in furthering our understanding of the genetic causation of disease.

The role of CNV variation in screening is presently less clear: one CNV associated with autism spectrum disorders (ASD) was studied by Kyle Walsh, my former graduate student. Autism is known to run in families, but the genetic origins are unexplained in 9 out of 10 people. One site, on chromosome 16 (p11.2), has been widely studied and is known to have deletions and duplications associated with autism, there being an approximately twenty-fold increase in risk with the duplication and a forty-fold increased risk with the deletion at 16 p11.2. What Kyle Walsh confirmed was that less than 1 percent of all ASD cases had this CNV, of either type, and that makes it a rather poor candidate for screening, even though it is so strongly associated with the disease.[9]

Gene-Environment Interaction and Disease

We have mentioned that some genetic variants may increase *susceptibility* to disease, but what does this mean? Unlike the complete chromosome additions and deletions, which guarantee a clinically bad outcome, the variant sometimes results in disease and sometimes does not. What makes the difference? In many cases, the influence of the gene depends on the environment. (It may also depend on the influence of other genes, but this is not considered further here.) *IL-4* is a gene that may have evolved to play a role in defending early primates against parasitic worms, but now some variations of it increase the risk of asthma if the person is exposed to dust mites and cockroaches. Of course, if a person is not exposed to mites and cockroaches the genetic variant cannot influence asthma risk. Susceptibility to asthma is conferred by the genetic variant but whether asthma materializes depends on there being environmental exposure. This is called a gene-environment interaction, and current research is starting to reveal many examples. The genetic variant may be a SNP or a CNV polymorphism, and numerous environmental agents are involved. Here are some examples.

Addiction is one of the scourges of modern life, and for most people this is not to cocaine, heroin, or any other illegal drug but to nicotine, alcohol, and perhaps to a lesser extent caffeine. Several genetic variations have now been shown to influence dependency on these substances, as well as on illicit drugs. One of the key factors is how quickly these substances are metabolized, and this is also under genetic control. People who are slow to metabolize alcohol are much less likely to continue drinking and as a consequence, not to suffer liver disease or other bad health effects from high alcohol consumption compared with rapid alcohol metabolizers. Heavy smoking increases the risk for all the smoking-related illness more than does light or no smoking, and here too genetic variation that influences nicotine addiction plays a role. For all these drugs, genes influence how much is consumed, how much stays in the body, and the risk of health effects from exposure. Each stage may be influenced by a different array of genes or different SNP variants within the same gene.

One gene, *CYP1A2*, wields a very strong influence on drug metabolism, including nicotine and caffeine, but the activity of this gene is speeded up by other environmental factors, including cigarette smoking and consumption of brassica vegetables (for example broccoli, cauliflower, cabbage). Other factors slow down *CYP1A2* activity, including apiaceous vegetables (for example, celery, parsnips, carrots), oral contraceptives, the luteal phase of the menstrual cycle, and theophylline used in bronchodilators. Pregnancy also influences drug metabolism; for many drugs this is slowed down as the pregnancy progresses. For example, the half-life of caffeine (how long it takes for blood levels of caffeine to be reduced by half) normally ranges from 2 to 4.5 hours, but by the end of pregnancy it is 12 to 18 hours.[10] Nicotine addiction is known to be influenced by social pressure to smoke, but individuals with a low genetic risk of smoking addiction have been shown to be more strongly influenced to smoke by their peers than are individuals whose dependency is more likely genetically determined.[11]

Environmental lead is a risk factor for poor fetal development, poor IQ, and low weight gain; however, variations in a gene that affects iron regulation, HFE, have also been shown to modify lead toxicity and its influence on infant birth weight. Studies of gene-environment interaction in pregnancy need to consider the genetic variations in both the mother and the fetus, and in this case, if the genetic variant occurred in either one, it modified the effect of lead on the child's birth weight.[12]

Elite athletes are not just the product of exercise. As many of us who are not so fit have suspected, there are also genetic variants that enhance athletic performance. A study of 700 British twin athletes found a link between athletic success and variants in the SLC9A9 gene, the same genetic region has also been associated with physical fitness.[13] Happiness is a trait that is influenced by both genes and gender, with genetic variants explaining 22 percent of heritability in males and almost double that in females, independent of other genes that influence depression.[14] Finally, in this eclectic group of studies demonstrating the wide range of environmental factors influencing genetic risk, it is established that risk of dental caries runs in families, but the risk of dental caries in primary and permanent teeth are influenced by different suites of genes.[15]

Epigenetic Causation

Jean-Baptiste Lamarck (1744–1829) was an eminent French biologist who made many early contributions to our understanding of natural history but whose legacy for the next 150 years was clouded by his theory of acquired traits. He believed that adaptations to the individual body could be passed on to the next generation. The example of this "baseless idea" that I was taught in my high school biology class was that if the sons of blacksmiths had strong arms and upper bodies, it was not because they had been inherited, as Lamarck would have it, but due to the environment in which they were brought up. However, we now know that DNA can acquire changes that are passed on to the next generation and, importantly, to subsequent generations. This is by a process called methylation, and the new science of these changes is known as epigenomics. It is pointing to new mechanisms for disease causation and also to novel methods for treating disease. Parenthetically, epigenomics has been used as a refutation of Darwinism, but it most decidedly is not (Darwin and Lamarck were friendly correspondents). Epigenomics is an alternative source of genetic variation that would not persist without the fundamental law of natural selection proposed by Darwin, who actually knew nothing about genetics. Variation produced by epigenetics, just like other genetic change, will not persist across generations unless the variants offer some survival advantage.

Epigenetics has been likened to computer software that uses the hardware of the less mutable DNA sequence. DNA molecules are supported by proteins, called "histones," which play a role in forming the structure of the chromosome. In recent years, it has been discovered that the histones serve other purposes and can exist in two essential states: acetylated, in which they serve to activate (switch on) a gene, or methylated, when the gene is deactivated. These changes do not alter the DNA sequence; rather, they function by changing gene expression, operating at the level of messenger RNA transcription in the manufacture of a protein. Messenger RNA (mRNA) carries genetic information from the DNA for the sequence of amino acids that will build proteins. Changing from one methylated state to the other is achieved by adding a methyl molecule to the histone, and that can be the result of changes to the diet.

Folic acid is an example of a powerful methylation agent. This may be one reason it is able, as a dietary supplement, to prevent the development of spina bifida. Epigenetic regulation now appears to be a powerful force in prenatal influences on later disease. Poor prenatal nutrition, such as occurs from being born during a famine, that is followed by overeating as a child is a very strong risk factor for the development of diabetes and a shorter life — and not just in the next generation but in the ones that follow. Epigenetic processes also affect mental illness. In a study of the Dutch population experiencing famine during World War II, poor maternal nutrition increased the risk of schizophrenia in offspring.

When epigenetic pathways are disrupted, genes may be activated or silenced. Almost every type of physical and mental illness is now being studied for epigenetic changes that may increase risk, and such changes are being found. The role of epigenetic change, just as with genetic effects, has been found to influence disease pathogenesis, progression, and severity. Epigenetic modification plays a role in every cancer in which it has been studied, in a large number of neurodegenerative conditions, in cardiovascular disease, and in autoimmune disorders. This area of research will almost certainly be highly productive over the next decades, and as it develops and just as happened with other genetic disease, the role of environmental risk factors and how they interact with epigenetic processes will require close scrutiny.[16]

Even though epigenetic changes are passed on in the DNA from one generation to the next, they are not irreversible, and this characteristic has resulted in the potential development of new therapies. Prostate, ovarian, lung, and melanoma cancers are all being actively studied for new therapies that target epigenetic processes underpinning the disease. In recent work from Brussels, breast cancers have been classified into estrogen positive and negative subtypes, and within these subtypes the epigenetic methylation profiles have been delineated with the anticipation of individualizing therapeutic options.[17]

Whether a mutation results in disease, and how severe that disease is, may also be influenced by which parent the mutation was inherited from. Prader-Willi syndrome (typically, small obese children with mild to moderate mental retardation) results from a deletion in chromosome 15 that always comes from the father. However, when the same deletion is inherited from the mother the child develops Angelman syndrome (severe mental retardation and the child has paroxysms of inappropriate laughing). The influence of high Immunoglobulin E on asthma risk is four times stronger if the mutation was derived from the mother, whereas a mutation in insulin growth factor 2 is active only if inherited from the father. In another study, the gene *Grb10* with an inactivated variant inherited from the father but not the mother resulted in more aggressive behavior in both male and female mice; humans also have this gene.[18] When Andre Agassi reportedly said, "I got a hundred bucks says my baby beats Pete's [Sampras] baby. I just think genetics are in my favor," he was surely thinking of the genetic contribution of Steffi Graf, their mother, more than his own!

Methodological Challenges and Opportunities

The genetic causation of disease is an extraordinarily complex area of research. Here are just three of the challenges. *Cryptic variation* is the difference in disease occurrence in people with the same mutation in one strand of the DNA because of variability in the healthy gene copy. *Allelic heterogeneity* occurs because several polymorphisms may be present in the same gene which requires that the SNP or CNV of interest must be specified, not just the gene. The *penetrance* of the gene may vary—this refers to the proportion of individuals that have the mutated gene that go on to develop the disease. For example, in early studies of BRCA1, 85 percent of the women with the disease variant developed breast cancer by age 70, but in the broader population this dropped (albeit still a very high risk) to 40 percent to 60 percent.

Mendelian Randomization

Finally, we should note that genetics offers a powerful tool for improving some of the research conducted to study harm (chapter 6). This new methodology examines individuals who carry the genetic variation that has been linked to the exposure. For example, low serum cholesterol has been associated with increased cancer risk. We know that many confounding factors and sources of bias must be controlled to confirm this association. But variations in the *APOE* gene have also been associated with low serum cholesterol, and if these same alleles are found to increase risk for cancer that would be powerful evidence in support of the hypothesized association. This is because the genetic variants can be assumed to have been randomly assorted at conception and so should be random with respect to all the co-variates that would normally need to be controlled if lipid levels themselves were being studied. This strategy has been called "Mendelian randomization" and it was used to powerful effect in a study to test the hypothesis that increased alcohol use decreases the risk of cardiovascular disease. In chapter 6, we discussed this problem and the difficulties of managing all the confounding factors linked to alcohol use.

Alcohol is metabolized by alcohol dehydrogenase, which is under the control of the *ADH3* gene, which has one or two copies of a polypeptide variant depending on whether the variant was inherited from one or both parents. Individuals with one variant copy clear alcohol more slowly than those without it and individuals with two copies more slowly still. The hypothesis was that persons with these variants would show correspondingly lower rates of heart disease because they should have higher blood alcohol levels. The result of the study confirmed the hypothesis. Among individuals consuming one or more drinks a day, those with one copy of the genetic variant had a 10 percent reduction in heart disease and those with two copies a 28 percent reduction compared to individuals with no copies of the variant. No effect of the genetic variant was seen in those drinking smaller amounts of alcohol. Since the genetic variants were randomly assorted, this study provides strong support for the protective effect of alcohol on cardiovascular disease.[19]

There is no doubt that variation in our genome is one of the most important and widespread causes of disease, almost certainly influencing every type of disease affecting humankind. Moreover, it is increasingly apparent that many of our personality traits, individual characteristics, and behaviors are also under considerable genetic control. The science of genetics has changed immeasurably over the last 20 years and is poised in the next 20 to profoundly add to our understanding of what causes disease and how. The challenges in this area of research are many, but they are being met with creativity, ingenuity, and excellent science. There is no area of studying disease causation that looks more promising.

ELEVEN

The Study of Mankind Is Man

Reflections on Animal Research

Experiments should be carried out on the human body. If the experiment
is carried out on the bodies of [other animals] it is possible that it might
fail for two reasons: the medicine might be hot compared to the human
body and be cold compared to the lion's body or the horse's body. . . .
The second reason is that the quality of the medicine might mean that
it would affect the human body differently from the animal body.
—Ibn Sina (c. 1012 CE). Kitab al-Qanun fi al-tibb,
Avicenna's Canon of Medicine

On Saturday, May 25, 1940, in Oxford at 11:00 a.m. Norman Heatley
administered a carefully measured dose of Streptomyces pyogenes to
eight white mice in what would become one of the most famous animal
experiments of all time. England was at war, and there were days when inva-
sion seemed imminent and bombing a certainty. Pristine college lawns had
been converted to growing vegetables, and the university was blacked out so
that no lights shone through the laboratory windows on South Parks Road.
At 12:00 noon two mice were given 5ml of penicillin Heatley had extracted
from mould juice, two mice received 10ml, and four were left untreated.
Over the next ten hours the first two mice received additional doses, and
then Heatley waited. He did not have to wait long. Thirteen hours after
starting the experiment, the first control mouse died; Heatley added a neat
red cross next to the animal's data in his laboratory notebook. Ninety minutes later two more control animals died, and the fourth two hours later.

Table 11.1 The First Animal Experiment
Using Penicillin, Saturday, May 25, 1940, Oxford

White Mice	11.00am Streptomyces pyogenes	Oxford 12.00 noon	2.15 pm	4.15 pm	6.20 pm	10.00 pm	Survival/ Death
			Penicillin Administered				
1	√	5ml	5ml	5ml	5ml	5ml	survived
2	√	5ml	5ml	5ml	5ml	5ml	13 d †
3	√	10ml					2 d †
4	√	10ml					6 d †
5	√	control					13 h †
6	√	control					14.5 h †
7	√	control					14.5 h †
8	√	control					16.5 h †

Source: Data reconstructed from Norman Heatley's laboratory notebook.

The first animal treated with penicillin died after two days, and two more six and thirteen days later. One survived. Clearly, Howard Florey, whose laboratory technician Heatley was, had produced an extract of penicillin that showed effectiveness in mice against this bacteria.

The first treatment of a patient with penicillin, at the Oxford Radcliffe Infirmary, to policeman Albert Alexander, was unsuccessful perhaps because of inadequate dosing. Penicillin was first successfully administered in America on March 14, 1942, at the Grace-New Haven Hospital to Anne Miller, the wife of Yale's athletic coach, who was near death from septicemia due to a beta-hemolytic streptococcus infection following a miscarriage. Mrs. Miller's physician, Dr. John Bumstead, was coincidentally treating Yale professor of physiology John Fulton for another bacterial infection acquired during a visit to a California laboratory. Knowing of Fulton's friendship with Florey—Fulton was caring for Florey's children in New Haven during the bombing blitz in England—Bumstead asked Fulton for assistance. This arrived in the form of 5.5 grams of pungent brown powder, mailed from the

Merck Pharmaceutical Company in New Jersey and representing half the total amount of penicillin then available in the United States. Florey and Heatley had visited the Merck Pharmaceutical Company executives to encourage them to start mass producing the drug, which they had just commenced. After some initial uncertainty as to how to prepare the drug and what dose to administer, Dr. Morris Tager injected 5,000 U every four hours starting at 4:00 p.m. Twelve hours later Mrs. Miller's temperature, which had spiked at 107°F, was normal, and she left hospital a few days later.

The initial mouse experiment was sufficiently compelling to move the research program forward, and it didn't require complicated statistical analysis because the results seemed obvious. Nor was penicillin ever put into clinical trials that for other drugs, despite their apparent efficacy, would be required today. The initial experimental and clinical experience, limited as it was, made the case for further use in humans. The development of penicillin is a scientific triumph of the first order, but its success was misleading with regards to being a model for drug development. There have been few other drugs that offered such a rapid and dramatic recovery. Moreover, penicillin was effective in both mice and man, which is not as common an occurrence as we would wish. Future drug discovery would have a more difficult road to follow.[1]

A thousand years after Ibn Sina expressed his reasoned opinion and a hundred after Alexander Pope's plea for secular understanding—"Know

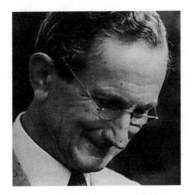

Figure 11.1. Dr. Norman Heatley OBE, 1911–2004.

then thyself, presume not God to scan; The proper study of Mankind is Man,"[2]—my colleagues and I attempted a formal examination of the frequency with which animal research was being systematically reviewed in the medical literature and how well. The results were disappointing: from the many million reports of animal experiments in the literature, we found only 25 systematic reviews of any specific topic and many problems with the methodological quality of animal research. We concluded that "much animal research into potential treatments for humans is wasted because it is poorly conducted and not evaluated in systematic reviews."[3]

Why does this matter? Most medical research is founded on animal experimentation: first a theoretical model is proposed, then some in vitro work at the molecular level might be conducted, onward to animal experiments, and then the first tests in humans with the large clinical trials being the definitive test. Harvard epidemiologist Walter Willett summed it up, "Those who practice epidemiology understand that the primary research mode is still the development of testable hypotheses based on sound biological reasoning."[4] But what if the biological reasoning is flawed and the animal research poorly conducted? Then the entire edifice of scientific research crumbles, patients are put at needless risk, and millions of research dollars are wasted. It is well recognized that as many as nine out of ten clinical trials fail to produce the expected positive results predicted by earlier experimental work, a state of affairs that jeopardizes the future of the pharmaceutical industry and the creation of new drugs. Observational studies are also known to frequently produce unreliable results (discussed in chapter 6).[5] But if implausible hypotheses are being propounded from flawed animal research, improvements in human research methods will not help, and this is another explanation for the failures of human research.[6]

A phase 1 trial was conducted at Northwick Park Hospital in West London of a monoclonal antibody TGN1412, which it was hoped could be used to treat leukemia and some of the autoimmune diseases. This was a "first-in-human" study, and six young healthy subjects volunteered for the treatment. The only previous subjects to receive this compound were animals including nonhuman primates (macaque monkeys), who were dosed at 500 times the amount subsequently administered to humans without producing any complications. The human trial results were disastrous. Despite being treated at doses many times lower than found to be safe in animals, all six volunteers suffered life-threatening toxicity and multiple organ failure and had to be admitted to intensive care. The animal experiments had failed utterly to predict what the response would be in humans.[7] Vaccine research also points to how poor animal models are for anticipating the human experience: not a single AIDS vaccine to date has proved effective in humans despite the apparent effectiveness of some 100 candidate vaccines studied in primates.

It has been known for many years that drug reactions in animals differ from those in humans, and some discrepancies have had tragic consequences. The sedative thalidomide (also discussed in chapter 6) was found to be safe in all animal species tested (except one variety of rabbit) and produced none of the limb malformations observed in human newborns. In contrast, steroids are broadly teratogenic in animals but not in humans. Not unexpectedly given the large number of animal studies conducted, some animal studies do predict human reactions quite well. We have seen that penicillin protected both mice and men from streptococcal infections and isotretinoin (the acne drug Accutane) causes birth defects in rabbits and monkeys (although not in mice or rats) as well as in humans. Some human carcinogens were predicted in animal studies (aflatoxins, benzene, diethylstilbestrol, vinyl chloride), but other agents were positive in animal but not in human studies (acrylamide, Alar, cyclamate, Red Dye #2, saccharin).[8] Owners of pets have sometimes found to their dismay that they cannot use the contents of their medicine cabinet to treat animals. Ibuprofen (Motrin) and aspirin can cause gastrointestinal ulceration and kidney damage in cats and dogs, and acetaminophen (Tylenol) is a poison to them.

Two principal reasons determine why animal research does not predict with any degree of certainty what the results will be in humans: methodology and metabolism. Methodologically poor research will always have problems being replicated, certainly across different species but also in experiments carried out in the same species. Moreover, if the experimental procedures are not fully reported, other investigators have no chance of accurately repeating the experiment. Pound et al. listed some of the major difficulties with animal research, and when studies have been done to reconcile differences between animal and human drug responses they invariably follow from one or more of these problems:

- Disparate animal species and strains, with a variety of metabolic pathways and drug metabolites, leading to variation in efficacy and toxicity

- Different models for inducing illness or injury with varying similarity to the human condition

- Variations in drug dosing schedules and regimen of uncertain relevance to the human condition

- Variability in animals for study, methods of randomization, choice of comparison therapy (none, placebo, vehicle)

- Small experimental groups with inadequate power, simple statistical analysis that does not account for confounding, and failure to follow intention to treat principles

- Nuances in laboratory technique that may influence results, for example, methods for blinding investigators, may be neither recognized nor reported

- Selection of outcome measures, may be disease surrogates or precursors, of uncertain relevance to the human clinical condition

- Length of follow up varies and may not correspond to disease latency in humans.[9]

The second major methodological difficulty with animal research is how rarely it is synthesized in a systematic way. The experience from studies of drugs to treat stroke is instructive. Hundreds of animal and human experiments have been conducted over decades of research in an attempt to find drugs that are effective in treating stroke. To date these have been strikingly unsuccessful, and in a major attempt to understand some of the reasons for this Malcolm Macleod, an Edinburgh neurologist, and colleagues have conducted some of the finest systematic reviews available in the experimental animal literature. In one systematic review of FK506 used for experimental stroke, in which 29 separate studies were found in the literature, major methodological errors were found: only 1 study blinded investigators to the drug intervention, only 2 blinded them for the outcome assessment, and none met all 10 study quality criteria established by the reviewers (1 study met none of the criteria and the highest score was 7). Meta-analysis of the animal FK506 studies demonstrated a strong trend for the methodologically weakest studies to show the strongest protective effects from the drug and the methodologically strongest studies to show no (or weak) protective effects.[10]

The quality of in vitro research and review, much of which is closely tied to animal experimentation, has been even less formally studied. In one rare example of how in vitro research is reviewed, a total of only 45 systematic reviews of any type of bench study was found in a literature that includes many millions of individual studies.[11] Even more alarming, Michael Rossner, executive editor of *The Journal of Cell Biology*, one of the most prestigious molecular biology journals, is reported as saying, "25% of all accepted manuscripts have had one or more illustrations that were manipulated in ways that violate the journal's guidelines," which included "photoshopping" to manipulate cell structures, and Ira Mellman, an editor of the same journal, noted, "In 1% of the cases we find authors have engaged in fraud."[12] It would be a mistake to exaggerate the extent of fraud in scientific research although it has been documented to occur: science is overwhelmingly a self-correcting discipline.

The poor quality of much animal and in vitro research poses substantial difficulty for researchers who use "biologic plausibility," one of the Bradford Hill criteria, as one of their guidelines for inferring causality (chapter 15). A discussion of biological mechanisms, usually relying on animal research, is ubiquitous in reporting clinical trials and in studies reporting epidemiological associations. However, the animal research on almost any topic of epidemiologic interest is so heterogeneous and inadequately synthesized that it is possible to selectively assemble a body of evidence from the animal and in vitro literature that will appear to support any epidemiologic result. Equally damaging to scientific productivity is the use of poorly synthesized and often biased reporting of the animal literature in grant applications. Major clinical trial programs are frequently launched in the absence of any systematic reviews of the supporting (and perhaps not so supportive) animal research. As clinical trials are launched to conduct the first large-scale testing of treatments in humans, the justification for them must rest almost entirely on in vitro studies and animal experiments. Neglecting to systematically review the relevant animal literature must, at least in part, explain the many human trials that fail to document effective and safe therapies.[13]

Publication bias is described elsewhere in this book as a major problem in reporting clinical trials and observational epidemiology (chapter 13). The proclivity for investigators to only write up their "positive" results and the preference of journal editors to publish them is well documented. But for many animal studies, usually conducted within a single laboratory and on a relatively small scale, how much more likely must be the opportunity for publication bias? It is difficult to hide a large multicenter trial that has involved numerous investigators, and the demand for trial registration has fortunately made trials even more transparent. But the lone researcher can readily run an experiment that did not turn out as hoped, and even though it might have been a valid study, the results never see the light of day. There has been little formal research into publication bias in in vitro or animal studies, and the few studies that have been reported find little evidence for bias, but given the enormous volume of animal research, this is hardly reassuring.[14] It seems likely that because of concern about proprietary information, much pharmaceutical animal research will remain unpublished, at least until the end of a research program, at which time it would have less value to other investigators. There is clearly enormous opportunity for substantial bias and misleading results in the animal literature used to create hypotheses that will be tested in human trials and epidemiological studies.

The discrepancy between the animal literature used to support trials and the corresponding trial results has been examined by Pablo Perel and colleagues from the London School of Hygiene and Tropical Medicine, who conducted systematic reviews of the animal and human studies in six clinical areas. A lack of consistency was shown in four of them. Corticosteroids have been shown to be ineffective in human head injury (discussed in chapter 5), but the animal studies showed a large improvement in functional recovery. Antifibrinolytics were successful in reducing bleeds in human trials, but the animal work was inconclusive. Tirilazad worsened the outcome for patients with ischemic stroke, but in animals it reduced the stroke area in the brain and improved functional outcomes. Steroids given before preterm birth in humans improved survival and reduced risk of respiratory distress, but in animals there was no clear decrease in mortality. Two areas where the human and animal research agreed were in the protective effects of tPA after ischemic stroke and the administration of bisphosphonates to increase bone mineral density.[15] What this research cannot show is whether the systematic reviews of the human or the animal literature were influenced by publication and other sources of bias, or if they reflect biological differences among species.

The use of animals for experimental research has raised ethical concerns in its own right. Opinions range from a view that no animal experimental work is ever justified, to an opinion that "it depends on the animal," which would rule out all experiments on primates and perhaps other higher species, to the other end of the spectrum and an argument that all animal research can be justified if done humanely. The current state of animal research suggests that much of it is wastefully repetitive and too often methodologically flawed, a situation that surely no legitimate scientist would wish to support. There is an urgent need to test animal models for their validity and their generalizability to the human condition, and to maintain updated systematic reviews of the animal evidence on a research topic as it accumulates. As necessary as humane animal research may be, it cannot be justified unless these other criteria are met.

An example of wasteful research was demonstrated by Emily Sena and colleagues at the University of Edinburgh, who have shown how animal research documenting the efficacy of tissue plasminogen activator (tPA) to treat stroke accumulated in the medical literature (figure 11.2). Overall, 450 experiments were done using a total of 5,262 animals, and except for the first year of research, there was never a time when the totality of evidence did *not* support a conclusion that tPA was an effective therapy in animals. By 1998, this was rigorously documented, and yet a decade of research

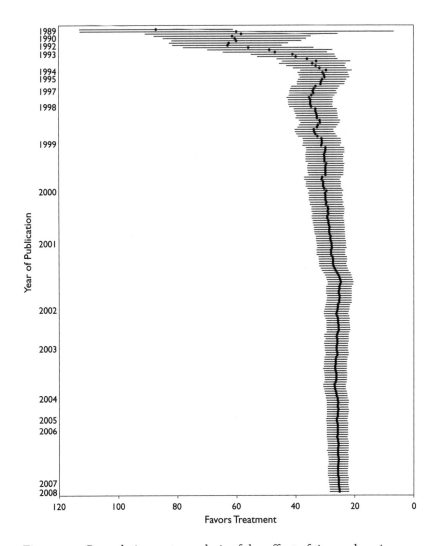

Figure 11.2. Cumulative meta-analysis of the effect of tissue plasminogen activator in (animal studies of) thrombotic occlusion models of stroke. Reprinted by permission from Macmillan Publishers Ltd: Sena ES, Briscoe CL, Howells DW, Donnan GA, Sandercock PA, Macleod MR. Factors affecting the apparent efficacy and safety of tissue plasminogen activator in thrombotic occlusion models of stroke: systematic review and meta-analysis. *J Cereb Blood Flow Metab.* 2010;30(12):1905–1913. Copyright 2010.

followed, with several thousand animals being given a stroke unnecessarily while the treatment was being repeatedly tested, with no additional benefit to knowledge.[16]

In 2010 the United Kingdom National Centre for the Replacement, Refinement and Reduction of Animals in Research published the ARRIVE guidelines (animal research: reporting in vivo experiments), which set criteria for publishing the details of the methods used in animal research. This included details of the animals used (species, strain, gender, developmental stage, weight, and source), husbandry and housing, sample size, how animals were allocated to experimental groups, definitions of study outcomes, and full reporting details of the results.[17] It was hoped that setting publication guidelines would lead to improvements in how the experiments were conducted; even more direct recommendations for conducting research were published by a European group of researchers.[18] While both of these represent important steps to improving the quality of animal research, reducing wasteful and unnecessary use of animals, and perhaps making it more easy to synthesize the results of repeated experiments, they do not address the other reasons for the poor predictability of the results of animal studies to what may be expected in humans. Even the better designed and conducted animal experiments are sometimes quite misleading.

How well do animal studies predict what will be observed in human studies? Here we must be careful to clarify what we mean by "predict." Just because some species of animal, out of a large number studied, have the same result as found in human research does not mean the criteria for prediction has been met. If enough experiments are done in many animal species, some will exhibit similar associations to humans just by chance. It is said that there are 40 million students of classical piano in China, in which case some brilliant concert pianists will inevitably be produced, irrespective of particular parenting styles and practice habits, that western Europeans frequently use to explain this success.

Prediction is at the heart of the scientific enterprise; it requires a specified hypothesis, in this case that a particular animal species and humans, because of some prejudged similarities, will react in the same way. Until 2005, the United States Environmental Protection Agency (EPA) judged that any chemical that appeared to be carcinogenic in *any* animal species, in just one study, was a "possible human carcinogen": "This group [possible human carcinogen] is used for agents with limited evidence of carcinogenicity in animals in the absence of human data. It includes a wide variety of evidence, e.g., (a) a malignant tumor response in a single well-conducted experiment that does not meet conditions for sufficient evidence, (b) tumor responses of marginal statistical significance in studies having inadequate design or reporting, (c) benign but not malignant tumors with an agent showing no response in a variety of short-term tests for mutagenicity, and (d) responses of marginal statistical significance in a tissue known to have a high or variable background rate."[19]

This liberal definition is quite easily met when one considers that animal studies could use extraordinarily high doses or could test dozens of species to find one that responded with a cancer, there was no human data, methodologically poor studies were counted, benign tumors counted, there was no need for rigorous statistical testing and no call for study replication. Little wonder, then, that hundreds of chemicals and drugs were considered possible human carcinogens. The use of such a loose criterion, based entirely on animal research, has had profoundly negative effects by adding costs to industry, prompting needless litigation, and leading to unnecessary worry for the public. It is notable that another organization that ranks chemicals for their carcinogenic risk, the International Agency for Research on Cancer (IARC), is much less likely than the EPA to determine a chemical as being a risk to humans.[20]

The confusion about prediction and association is further demonstrated by the American Cancer Society's statement about animal research, below.[21]

> Although it isn't possible to predict with certainty which substances will cause cancer in humans based on lab studies alone, virtually all known human carcinogens that have been adequately tested produce cancer in lab animals. In many cases, carcinogens are first found to cause cancer in lab animals and are later found to cause cancer in people.

But for safety reasons, it is usually assumed that exposures that cause cancer at larger doses in animals may also cause cancer in people. It isn't always possible to know the relationship between exposure dose and risk, but it is reasonable for public health purposes to assume that lowering human exposure will reduce risk.[22]

We saw in chapter 7 that the correct way to analyze data that is used to predict a disease or a diagnosis is to estimate the true and false positive and the true and false negative results. What the ACS doesn't consider is how many substances were found carcinogenic in animal studies but not in humans, how many species were involved, how many studies were done, and what dose levels were tested.

These types of linkages are not evidence of predictability, a topic discussed by Niall Shanks and colleagues who describe toxicology tests that show predictive values from animal to human response that are no better than a coin toss;[23] moreover, the tests were for a positive result in humans as well as in *any* animal species of all those tested, which further increased the opportunity for a chance result.

Genetic studies are conducted in a whole range of animal species, including some very primitive ones: fruit flies, flat worms, and bacteria. We discussed in chapter 10 how inter-individual genetic variation is so important in determining drug reactions among humans, and so it should not be surprising to learn that this heterogeneity is even greater among different animal species. It is important to remember that our genome is a dynamic structure extending back to the very first replicating DNA in some warm pool on a highly volcanic planet. As Allan Spradling from the Howard Hughes Medical Institute puts it, "Current species and genomes represent only a snapshot in the continuum of now extinct forms, adapted to now extinct environments, stretching back to the first groupings of biomolecules on the young earth."[24]

It has become increasingly obvious over decades of molecular genetic research that our genome has conserved much of the function of earlier genomes; evolution reuses older structures in novel ways rather than creating entirely new forms. This means there will be commonality in genetic function among species, but most of it is not presently understood: some details of genetic expression are emerging, but the task of specifying expression in a single gene, let alone thousands of genes, or in tens of thousands of genetic interactions has barely started. Homologies occur throughout biology, the same structure having evolved to serve different functions—bird wings and our forearm being the archetypical example—and these are increasingly recognized throughout the human genome; suites of genes evolved for one purpose are subsequently adopted for others.

Does this mean that genetic function observed in animal studies will predict what occurs in humans? Will clone creation, genetic engineering, stem cell research, pharmacogenomic studies, and all the other research endeavors where animal genomics are investigated provide clues as to what to expect in humans? Clues, most probably; accurate prediction, almost certainly not: animal research is crucial for creating leads and hypotheses for human genomic research, but it will never be a substitute for human investigation. Genes function inside the internal environment of a complex organism (the cell and the body), and the organism in turn must survive in complex external environments. As these change so may the functionality of a gene. The low predictive power of genetic studies is little different from the fallibility of all animal research in trying to predict drug reactions; each genetic sequence will need to be tested in rigorously designed experiments to examine the utility of its expression and function when its role in developing future therapies is being considered.

TWELVE

Celebrity Trumps Science

It's the truth I'm after, and the truth never harmed anyone.
What harms us is to persist in self-deceit and ignorance.
—Marcus Aurelius. Meditations, Book 6, 21. Trans. Gregory Hayes, 2002

While I sat writing on a beautiful lakeside in Patagonia, the tranquility was shattered by the arrival of a crew filming a TV reality show, the name of which will remain anonymous to protect the guilty. The idea behind the show was unclear, but what we saw were several kayaks being paddled toward the beach where four large polystyrene figures had been erected. Mapuche idols, we were told, but they looked like a cross between Easter Island and the Northwest totems. The local Mapuche people, now generally well assimilated into modern Argentine life, would have been bewildered. After a leisurely break and with cameras rolling again the "castaways" ran off to a nearby hillside to encounter more "danger." It is hard to imagine a more unreal reality, but this is apparently what many people watch with pleasure. Perhaps no surprise, then, that credulous belief in manufactured adventure also leads to a ready acceptance of the belief that if disease appears to cluster around an environmental source, it must be caused by it. Especially if a celebrity says that it is so.

The world is so awash in false information, misleading advertising, and rank promotion that messages based on real evidence are drowned in a flood of untruths. The original guru of messaging, Marshall McLuhan, could not have envisaged a world where information arrives instantaneously, unedited, and is continuously at our fingertips in a flood of blogs, rants, tweets, and pop-ups, and where anyone can tout his or her recommendations and cures for all that ails us, and for much more that doesn't. How can the untrained recipient of this noise of Babel have any possible way of understanding that much of what is heard has never been validated, will likely be of absolutely no benefit, is going to waste money and time, and may be harmful? Some of the advertising is patently ridiculous, and one would hope that it is so to all but the most gullible. Let us first consider evening primrose oil and huperzine A (HupA).

Evening Primrose Oil

Five minutes on the Internet with the relevant search terms will turn up a plethora of websites advertising the benefits of evening primrose oil. "Essential fatty acids have many beneficial effects on the body and influence hormone production and immune and cardiovascular health," notes one of the more balanced claims (Solgar website, July 2011). The "Complimentary Medical Association" flatly states that primrose oil is being used to treat premenstrual syndrome, menstrual cramps, and rheumatoid arthritis. It cites a long list of references to the scientific literature (none more recent than 2003) and helpfully provides a link to a site to purchase the oil. Another website "Stylehive" tells that Kate Moss (a model) and Liv Tyler (an actress) use "Rodin's olio lusso," a compound containing the "miracle oil" as part of their "home mini peel." Here too a link to a sales site is provided.

Evening primrose oil has been studied in quite a number of clinical trials, although many of the trials are of generally poor methodological quality. The reports of most of them are unclear as to whether randomization was properly concealed and if the person assessing the effect of treatment was blind to therapy. The clinical trials have been systematically reviewed by authors from the Cochrane Collaboration. Here is a summary of their conclusions as of July 2011. Primrose oil used for preeclampsia—insufficient data and so unknown effectiveness; chronic fatigue syndrome—effectiveness unknown; breast pain—likely to be ineffective or harmful (in the United Kingdom the license was withdrawn for this indication; it is astonishing that it was ever granted); rheumatoid arthritis—"there is insufficient evidence for any reliable assessment of efficacy to be made"; premenstrual syndrome—no evidence of benefit; multiple sclerosis—lack of evidence to support prophylactic use. Clearly, there is inadequate evidence to support any claims of benefit.

Based on a preliminary small randomized trial treating children who had developmental coordination disorder with a supplement containing 80 percent fish oil and 20 percent evening primrose oil (omega-3 and omega-6 oils, respectively) that showed some benefits in reading, spelling, and behavior, the Durham County Council in the United Kingdom took the giant leap of implementing a massive intervention "trial" among some 3,000 healthy teenage children. If this had been a properly randomized trial, it would have been a laudable effort, but sadly it was no such thing. This study has been the subject of much controversy, has never been published despite enormous media coverage, and only the investigative reporting of Ben Goldacre of the *Guardian* newspaper revealed that this was a fatally flawed study. All the Durham County Council websites for this study appear to have been deleted, and so the information discussed here comes second-hand from other media sources. This project was initially reported to be a "trial," which would lead one to expect that the children had been randomized to the supplement or placebo (an olive oil supplement has been found useful in this regard). In fact, there was no randomization. All the children were scheduled to receive the omega oils.

A requirement for conducting randomized trials is that the investigators must be uncertain as to the benefit and risks of the new therapy—a presumption known as "equipoise." However, the leading investigators in Durham reflected no uncertainty. Dave Ford, the chief inspector of schools, was reported in the *Daily Mail* as saying, "We don't see this as an experiment, we really believe that this is going to work," and Dr. Madelaine Portwood, the senior educational psychologist, in the same newspaper, "Previous trials have shown remarkable results and I am confident that we will see marked benefits in this one as well." This lack of objectivity may explain why no control group was used in this study, why an opportunity for good science to actually examine the effectiveness and safety of the supplement in normal children was missed, and why the participants of this trial were not able to contribute to scientific knowledge.

Using freedom of information requests, Goldacre was able to secure, from the Durham Council's reluctant grasp, some details of the study that had not been previously released. He writes that of the initial 3,000 or more children originally entered in the study, only about a quarter (832) maintained 80 percent compliance with the supplement regimen by the end of the study. From these, 629 compliant children (what happened to the other 203 of them?) were then "matched" against 629 non-supplement takers. School performance was reported to be better among the supplement takers, which is entirely predictable. This is an incorrect procedure for analyzing these data, and readers of this book will now appreciate that another fundamental problem has occurred. Given the lack of a properly randomized control group, the study cannot avoid selection bias (described in chapter 6) whereby those children who are compliant in taking their pill regimen are also highly likely to be more compliant in doing their homework, completing reading assignments, and participating in other educational activities that will improve their school performance. Because of this, their success cannot be attributed to the omega supplement.

Importantly, and in a clear violation of medical ethics, there also appears to have been no attempt to document any complications that may occur from using evening primrose oil. Some of the side effects from fatty acids that should have been inquired about concern possible blood thinning leading to nose bleeds, diarrhea, and risk of increased mercury levels. Other possible complications relate to the oxidation of fatty acids, which can produce free radicals with the potential to increase the risk of cancer and degenerative diseases. So-called natural supplements are far from free of possible side effects, and reporting them should be part of any trial of supplements.[1]

HupA

There are numerous "celebrity doctors" who promote their newsletters and books online. One is a Dr. Mark Stengler, whose summer 2011 newsletter "Bottom Line Natural Healing," which can be purchased for $7.95, had a front-page story: "Forbidden herbal cures—proven effective in hundreds of studies . . . yet supplement makers are prohibited by law from telling you about them." This story was about huperzine A (HupA), an extract of Chinese club moss. Dr. Stengler tells his readers that HupA "boosts your levels of acetycholine" just as do the Alzheimer's drugs Aricept and Cognex, except that "HupA is a lot safer." He mentions "studies" that show HupA works better than the conventional drugs, protects the brain from free radical damage, increases blood flow better than ginkgo, and reduces the formation of beta-amyloid. We are told that "these benefits are unprecedented in the history of medical science" and that most people have never heard of HupA because "according to the Dietary Supplement Health Education Act of 1994, supplement makers are forbidden from claiming that any of their products can cure or even prevent disease!" Then the coup de grâce: "Luckily, I'm a doctor and not a supplement manufacturer. That means that I'm free to tell you the whole truth about the healing power of vitamins, herbs, and other supplements."

What does the evidence from randomized clinical trials tell us about HupA and Alzheimer's disease? (Chapter 5 emphasized that randomized trials are the only valid way of establishing the effectiveness for any therapy.) In the PubMed database organized by the US National Library of Medicine, which contains more than 20 million records and is the most comprehensive database of medical research anywhere, eight clinical trials that studied HupA were listed (accessed July 7, 2011). Six trials were from China, and three of these were published in Chinese. Their English abstracts suggest positive results, but the trials are all very small and without a valid translation there is no way of knowing whether correct trial procedures were followed. The other three Chinese trials were published in English and include two very small trials indicating some clinical benefit and one trial that compared two methods of administering HupA and so it was unable to assess HupA's efficacy.

Of the two studies from the United States, one was a pharmacokinetic study that did not address any clinical outcomes and the other was a phase 2 trial (described in chapter 5) testing the efficacy of HupA in mild to moderate Alzheimer's disease. It concluded: "This study provides Class III evidence [that means it came from a randomized controlled trial] that huperazine A 200 μg BID [the abbreviation pharmacists unhelpfully use for 'bis in die' —

Latin for twice a day] has no demonstrable cognitive effect in patients with mild to moderate AD." All told, this is far from compelling evidence that HupA has any beneficial effects. The Dietary Supplement Act of 1994 did have a purpose. The promotion of vitamins and supplements is not a harmless occupation. If patients choose to use them in preference to clinically proven safe and effective therapies, they are unwittingly putting themselves at risk of potentially harmful complications, of increasing the progression and severity of their disease, and of dying.[2]

But we are all potential victims; the Yale Alumni Magazine, with its well-educated readership, for months ran an advertisement for unscented formulas of pheromones that would increase "affection" for men and women. Two very specific citations to *Time* and *Newsweek* were provided, but there was only vague reference to "two 8 week double-blind studies." Joseph of Michigan certainly approved, stating that "the affection level went up 20 fold," but what did the actual studies show? A search of PubMed turned up the two mentioned studies.[3] In the study of women, 19 received the pheromone added to a fragrance and 17 received a placebo that they used for six weeks. The investigators looked at changes in the individual's own behavior measured by: petting/kissing/affection, sleeping next to romantic partner, sexual intercourse, formal dates, informal dates, male approaches, and masturbation, based on a prior two-week baseline period. The major difficulties in this research are the small sample size and the short baseline period, one that can hardly produce valid estimates of "normal" behavior. Indeed, of the measures that appeared to improve after pheromone use (the first four in the list), three were lower in the pheromone group at baseline. What is being observed is most likely a regression to the mean effect (chapter 8). The study of males was similarly small and had the same design, but in this one, apparently ignored by the advertisement, affection was not improved after pheromone treatment (both studies discussed their findings in terms of "attractiveness," quite a different concept from the "affection" being promised in the advertisement). There were major differences in the number married versus not, and those who were dating versus not, in the pheromone and control groups, which could substantially influence the results. One has to conclude that both studies have been grossly overinterpreted, and it cannot go unremarked that the pheromone study results were intended for market-ing, and marketed they surely were.

Advertisements for health elixirs are probably as old as the first cities: the ancient Roman's favorite condiment garum, a pungent fish sauce, was widely promoted: "Scaurus' tunny jelly, blossom brand, put up by Euty-ches, Slave of Scaurus,"[4] and just as today, products promoting hair growth, virility, and longevity prevailed in the ancient world. The claims of Pompe-ian graffito could happily compete on the walls of any modern city.

Paradoxically, in spite of the widespread public suspicion over phar-maceutical company advertising, it is among the most reliable sources of health information about health products available to the public. Drug ad-vertising is highly regulated by the US Food and Drug Administration, and while there is often a constant tug of war between a company's marketing divisions, its regulatory affairs division, and the company scientists, the most egregious claims, which are common for non-pharmaceutical products, are generally avoided in pharmaceutical drug advertising.[5]

Self-promotion is not regulated, and anyone is free to recommend her fa-vorite potion, behavioral modification, dietary supplement, and weight-loss technique as numerous shelves in the health section of any bookstore and a plethora of online advertising will attest. How can the producers of properly validated studies, such as the Cochrane Collaboration's systematic reviews, hope to compete in such a free market place of opinion? To aggravate the problem, this is a public that has rarely benefited from even the slightest whiff of any exposure to science during their formal education, and it is ill equipped to evaluate the rabid claims it encounters daily. In the United States, some children are not even educated in the theory of evolution and so can have no understanding of modern biology and, ipso facto, have no hope of understanding matters of evidence and causality. They have been left exposed to medieval quackery and paleolithic shamanism, however much dressed in modern guise.

To make matters worse, numerous nonvalidated claims are promoted, and science-supported research decried, by celebrities who feel the need, and are often handsomely paid, to impose their own strongly (or perhaps not) held beliefs on the rest of us. This is despite their not having a shred of expertise in the science arenas into which they happily plunge, and with no apparent concern about the unintended consequences of what they are promoting.

My first personal experience of this put me up against Paul McCartney and Joanna Lumley, two people I greatly admire for, respectively, their music and their comedy. I did not fare well. It started with a telephone call from the producers of a TV science show produced in Britain, who wanted to film an interview with me about research I had recently published suggesting an increased risk for low birth weight babies among mothers who smoked marijuana during their pregnancy. This film was intended to be a story about drug use among British youth and included other health effect work, including a suggested increased risk of lung cancer from marijuana smoke. When the film was shown, I watched it with my two children and was bemused by two included interviews, one with McCartney and the other with Lumley, who both, without providing any contrary scientific evidence, mocked the research shown on the show and observed they did not see any problems with marijuana use. My children's reaction was swift: "Dad, you lost," and they were right; but the main losers were the children of mothers who might have been persuaded to think twice about continuing their marijuana habit during pregnancy. With that audience, the white coats stood slim chance against a rock star and a brilliant comedienne.

Meryl Streep is one of the world's finest actresses, but she doesn't have a lot of experience in environmental science. That didn't stop her campaigning vigorously to ban Alar, a chemical used to prevent rot on apples. Despite the lack of any scientific evidence that Alar caused health effects, it became a cause célèbre for a host of celebrities. Surely the consequences were unintended: some apple farmers were put out of business, migrant workers lost their jobs, and apples became so scarce that eating "an apple a day to keep the doctor away" became impossible. Nor was this a time to encourage apple eating for school lunches.

F. Peter Guengerich, a distinguished biochemist and toxicologist at Vanderbilt University, has probably never met Arnold Schwarzenegger, a former weight lifter and actor, but their opposing views on phthalates, used as plastic softeners, were featured by the American Council on Science and Health, an organization promoting science-based public policy.[6] Schwarzenegger, who was governor of California at the time, confidently proclaimed, "these chemicals threaten the health and safety of our children," while Professor Guengerich could only reply that, based on over one thousand research publications, the evidence showed that phthalates did not pose a risk to humans. You would think there was no contest in the weight of evidence and you would be right, but not in the way expected. Phthalates have been banned in numerous states, with no evidence of any benefit to health. The plastics industry has incurred considerable additional expense, the cost of which cannot be simply passed on to customers.

Actor Steve McQueen promoted the use of Laetrile, a drug derived from apricot pits, administered in Mexican clinics to treat cancer without any evidence from clinical trials that it was effective. McQueen went to Mexico in 1980 for treatment of a rare cancer, but his praise for Laetrile as a wonder drug was somewhat undermined by his dying a few months after starting treatment. When Laetrile was put into clinical trials at Sloane Kettering Memorial Hospital in New York it was found unequivocally to have no benefit. Unusually, these trials were based not on sound pharmacological evidence but rather to convince patients they should not abandon recommended medical therapy to travel to Mexico.

Celebrities have always lent their names to product promotion. Cigarette manufacturers employed the biggest movie stars of the day to promote their lethal products: Joan Fontaine for Chesterfield along with actor Ronald Reagan "I'm sending Chesterfields to all my friends. That's the merriest Christmas any smoker can have." Basil Rathbone helped sell Fatima cigarettes and Al Jolson sold Lucky Strike: "It's toasted. No throat irritation—no cough," as he was a singer we should hope that was true. United States Senator Robert Dole's long political career ended courageously with his sensitive promotion of the erectile dysfunction drug Viagra, a product that does work. It would be reassuring to believe that celebrities really investigated the validity behind the product claims that they tout, but one has to suspect it is the financial contract that may benefit from the most scrutiny.

No higher authority than His Royal Highness Prince Charles of the British royal family has opined on the effectiveness of alternative medicine:

"The proper mix of proven complementary, traditional and modern remedies, which emphasizes the active participation of the patient, can help to create a powerful healing force in the world." He added, "Many of today's complementary therapies are rooted in ancient traditions that intuitively understood the need to maintain balance and harmony with our minds, bodies and the natural world." "Much of this knowledge, often based on oral traditions, is sadly being lost, yet orthodox medicine has so much to learn from it." If this were a call for more research into the effectiveness and safety of alternative therapies, it would be welcome, but Prince Charles simply states as a fact that alternative therapies are beneficial. In fact, many clinical trials have been done, although often of poor quality, to test several alternative therapies, and the results are not encouraging. The better the quality of the trial, the less likely it is that any benefit is shown. My own skepticism was aroused on a visit to an acupuncture clinic at the leading Beijing hospital in 1982 where every possible ailment was being treated by acupuncture. A patient with a grossly protruding eye, suspicious of a massive brain tumor, did not look like a promising candidate for the acupuncture he was being given, and reports of the use of acupuncture as an anesthetic for open-heart surgery were truly alarming.

The Cochrane Library accessed (January 27, 2011) for the systematic reviews of *Ginkgo biloba* showed no evidence of benefit for leg muscle pain (intermittent claudication—based on 14 trials), or for tinnitus (3 trials), cognitive impairment and dementia (36 trials), adult macular degeneration (2 trials), and stroke (10 trials). For acupuncture the results are equally discouraging, with even more trials providing no evidence of benefit observed for: cancer pain, chronic asthma, cocaine dependence, glaucoma, schizophrenia, depression, Bell's palsy, insomnia, epilepsy, and acute stroke. There was limited evidence of benefit for: tension headache, menstrual pain (primary dysmenorrhea), pain from labor induction, and, perhaps most convincingly, migraine. The results are equally not very encouraging for other alternate therapies. The onus is on the many believers in alternative therapy, which is a multibillion-dollar annual business that frequently benefits from celebrity endorsement, to validate their claims. Perhaps Prince Charles is right and orthodox medicine can learn from the unorthodox, but the first lessons must go in the other direction; unorthodox medicine must allow itself to be validated using appropriate clinical testing. If its therapies are shown to be effective and safe, they will surely be quickly adopted into modern medicine.

Although some might shudder at the prospect, the leaders of the Christian churches are among the greatest celebrities of our time. Except for the Jehovah's Witnesses, who have a wanton disregard for the well-being of their children and relatives, most Christian leaders recommend that their adherents follow modern medicine and accept therapeutic interventions. But they also practice their own particular therapeutic maneuver. It is called "intercessory prayer" and is directed to their God to request the recovery to good health for themselves and others, apparently without pondering why God allowed the illness in the first instance. But what is the evidence that prayer has any effect? Unlike praying for one's own health, which might be studied using psychological paradigms of motivation, esteem, and the placebo effect, praying for others can be studied using formal clinical trial methods. The study design is not difficult: a series of patients with similar illnesses are randomly allocated so that half receive the benefit of prayer from appropriate worthies who are well versed in what it takes to make a strong prayer. Patients from the other half are left alone to their own prayers and to the prayers of those who might normally pray for them. If the trial has a large enough number of people and is conducted in a rigorous way, it would be a fair test of the benefit of the additional intercessory prayers. Has such a trial been done? It seems obvious that no church would advocate for this type of a trial, arguing instead that faith is so strong that a trial would be redundant. However, if faith was so strong that it was thought that a trial could document an effect of prayer, even if just to convince those of us who are less confident, then a trial would surely have been done a long time ago.

Ten randomized prayer trials, which included a total of 7,646 patients, have been conducted by scientists. For some patients, a God was petitioned in addition to them receiving standard care, compared to a control group of patients that received only standard care. The systematic review authors conclude that there is no evidence that intercessory prayer showed any benefit. To their credit, and unlike almost any other group of scientists who always suggest more research would be important, they also conclude: "We are not convinced that further trials of this intervention should be undertaken and would prefer to see any resources available for such a trial used to investigate other questions in health care."[7] To which one can only add "amen."

Jenny McCarthy is a former *Playboy* playmate of the year, model, and actress, but she is perhaps best known for her prominent role as an activist, claiming that childhood vaccines can cause autism. She has played a leading role in organizations that condemn vaccination, has authored a book on the topic, and is a frequent guest on talk shows commenting on vaccine safety. Her activism started after her son was diagnosed with autism (although some experts have said his symptoms suggest Landau-Kleffner syndrome, with which autism can be misdiagnosed). In fact, there is no evidence to support a role of vaccines in autism; initially it was claimed that thimerosal, a preservative used in some vaccines, was the responsible agent, but after this was removed from vaccines, there was no observable reduction in autism incidence. Recently claims have been made about other ingredients and the number of vaccinations being given, all of which are entirely speculative.

The link between the MMR vaccine (measles-mumps-rubella) administered to young children and autism was first suggested by Andrew Wakefield and colleagues in a 1998 paper in the *Lancet*. As soon as it was published, this paper was controversial and methodologically suspect. It was eventually found to be fraudulent and has now been retracted.[8] Wakefield was struck off the British list of practicing doctors. Jenny McCarthy's response was to blame the people who questioned and investigated Wakefield's research. McCarthy has also promoted chelation therapy as a cure for autism, a procedure for which there is no evidence of benefit.

Unfortunately, the celebrity led anti-vaccination campaign has resulted in immunization rates of only 80 percent in the United Kingdom and closer to 60 percent in some parts of the United States, well below the 90 percent vaccination rate needed to protect all children in the community (this is called "herd immunity"). Substantial increases in disease have followed, including an epidemic of measles in the United Kingdom, where measles cases rose from 70 in 2001 to 1,143 in 2009. With a case fatality rate of around two per thousand cases, deaths have resulted from the anti-vaccine campaign. There have been other consequences; there are about 200,000 deaths annually worldwide from measles, and attempts to eradicate the disease have been thwarted, hopefully temporarily.

Autism is a very difficult disease to diagnose, and the diagnosis has changed in recent years to include a spectrum of disorders that were not previously included in the diagnosis. Adding to the conditions that qualify as autism spectrum disorder must inevitably increase the incidence of the disease. If autism really is on the rise, this cannot be entirely due to genetic causes—genes do not mutate that quickly. Rather, a real increase would point to a new environmental agent. Research into other causes of autism has been distracted by the vaccine controversy. Of course, genetic causes are also being explored, and these are likely to be where the first breakthroughs occur.

Celebrity comments are not always met with approval and agreement. In September 2011, Michele Bachmann, a sometime Republican candidate for the U.S. presidency asserted, in a much-publicized remark, that the vaccine given to 11- or 12-year-old girls to prevent infection by the human papilloma virus (HPV) resulted in "mental retardation" (using, to add insult to injury, a now disused and widely considered insulting term). HPV is a cause of seven out of ten cervical cancers and nine out of ten cases of genital warts. Over 20 million people in the United States are infected with HPV, and each year 12,000 women are diagnosed with cervical cancer and 4,000 die from the disease. Bachmann's statement was not even based on any self-belief; rather, she was repeating what she had heard from a woman she had just met in a crowd of well-wishers. According to an Institute of Medicine Report published just one month previously, over 35 million doses of HPV vaccine had been administered without evidence of it causing any neurological or other similar conditions.[9] Although Bachmann's remark was met with widespread and fully deserved opprobrium, one pediatrician commented that she was likely to be dealing with unnecessary worry about the HPV vaccine long after the candidate had been forgotten. In November 2011, a task force in the United States recommended extending the HPV vaccine to young boys.

The influence of celebrity can have such a negative impact on the public's understanding of disease causation and on how scientists try to uncover the causes of disease. Celebrities would not have much influence without media promotion, and while there are some responsible health and medical journalists, there are many more who fail to provide a balanced view. The Internet is increasingly the principal source of health news for many people, but it is completely uncontrolled and often lacks any responsible editorial balance. Trolling through Internet sites while exploring the Jenny McCarthy episode was a revelation of the extreme positions taken by both sides of the strident vaccine debate. When the public is so poorly prepared to understand the science underlying health debates, it is vulnerable to celebrity exploitation. But how much does celebrity behavior and practice influence people? Is there more to it than the public's inability to understand scientific concepts? There is surprisingly little empirical research on the influence of celebrity, but that which has been done suggests that celebrities are indeed influential. Some of the key conclusions follow, but in a book that emphasizes the precepts of evidence-based medicine, it should be pointed out that there appear to be no clinical trials in this area, though designing them would not be especially difficult, and that the papers in the literature may be subject to publication bias.

Former First Lady Nancy Reagan had a mastectomy rather than breast conserving surgery (BCS) in October 1987. A database of more than 160,000 women diagnosed with breast cancer indicated that there was a 25 percent decline in BCS during the next six months, with a return to normal rates after that.[10] Another area of public health concern has been the influence of movie stars smoking on the screen on the initiation of smoking in adolescents. In one study, nonsmoking adolescents named their favorite film stars, whose films were then studied to quantify the amount they smoked. Adolescents whose favorite film star was an onscreen smoker were more likely to become smokers themselves.[11]

Mark McGwire, who held the single-season record for home runs in baseball, until surpassed by Barry Bonds three years later, has been associated with two public health problems: positively, supporting child abuse prevention programs and, negatively, the use of the muscle-building supplement Androstenedione. His influence on both topics was found to be substantial in both the public's attitude toward child abuse and regarding use of the supplement.[12] Celebrity can even influence suicide: when the famous male television actor M. J. Nee hanged himself in Taiwan, in the following month there was a substantial increase in the number of suicides, particularly in suicide by hanging. The age group affected was younger than the dead celebrity and presumably more impressionable.[13]

The influence of celebrities in health messaging is very apparent. They can be a force for good or they can significantly undermine the success of beneficial health messages. Not surprisingly, many celebrities become involved in their "causes" because of personal involvement: a sick parent, spouse, or child. One can only hope that with an awareness of their powerful ability to influence the public, celebrities will seek help in determining what the scientific basis is for their claims. On the other hand, if modern celebrities adopted the less angst ridden views of Oscar Wilde, a nineteenth-century celebrity, they would pose much less of a problem for the rest of us. Wilde is known for the remark: "To get back my youth I would do anything in the world, except take exercise, get up early or be respectable."

THIRTEEN

Replication and Pooling

The criterion of the scientific status of a theory is its
falsifiability, or refutability, or testability.
—*Karl R. Popper, 1963*

No trial is an island, entire of itself; every trial is a
piece of the continent, a part of the main.
—*Mike Clarke and Iain Chalmers, 1998, paraphrasing Donne, 1623*

To Karl Popper, one of the most influential philosophers of science of the twentieth century, verification and falsifiability were central to the scientific enterprise. It was, he thought, only through replication that the truthfulness of a scientific observation could be assured or rejected. There are two types of replication. One seeks to replicate everything in the original experiment: the study participants, what was done to them, and which study outcome is assessed. All are repeated in the second experiment to see if the same result ensues. The second type of replication varies the experimental condition, perhaps doing the experiment in a different gender, age group, or racial group. Each type of replication serves a different purpose. The first tests whether the initial experimental results are due to chance, the likelihood of which diminishes with each successful replication. The second type of replication is a deductive process whereby failure to replicate sets up alternative hypotheses: if the experiment produces a different result in, say, younger rather than older people, is there a plausible explanation for this that generates another hypothesis?[1]

In this chapter, we are largely concerned with using replication to rule out chance as an explanation for study results. New hypotheses are derived from many sources: from observations in the laboratory or in the clinic, by analogy from other data, as well as by failure to replicate an early study result. Validating a study result, through replication, must have priority if the scientific process is to move forward in an orderly and systematic fashion but also if clinical guidelines, legal opinions and public health policies are to be based on sound evidence.

Does replication mean exactly repeating the methods used in the previous experiments? Certainly not: if the first study was biased, perhaps the interviewers were not blinded to the case-control status of their interviewees, it would be foolish for the next study to make the same mistake. Replication should be a series of studies of ever-improving methodology as one learns from the previous mistakes. Where is all this reported? The systematic review, described more fully below, provides the basis for synthesizing existing evidence compiled from all the studies on a particular topic and, properly reviewed, will identify the methodological weaknesses of the past work and make recommendations for future studies. New studies are not just replicating the results of earlier research; rather, they should be based on all of the evidence to date. Moreover, when a new study has been completed, authors need to integrate their findings back to the totality of evidence, possibly through an updated statistical synthesis (meta-analysis) if that is warranted. As Clarke and Chalmers have so evocatively, with Donne's help, described it: no piece of research is an island unto itself and study results should not "be viewed in isolation from the whole body of relevant previous research"; they need to find their "continent."[2]

In a recent publication, in which my colleagues and I reported the association of a new gene PDE11A with atopic asthma, the paper included a replication in five other data sets from other research groups.[3] This reflects an emerging trend in reporting genetic studies that use a new technology called a genome-wide association study (GWAS) where between 100,000 to 1 million single nucleotide polymorphisms (SNPs) are examined for their association with a disease (see chapter 10 for more details). In traditional scientific reports, a paper is judged on the validity of its own methods, on the plausibility of the findings, and the study results are either replicated or not, as the case may be, in future papers by the same or other investigators. PDE11A, a recently identified gene in the phosphodiesterase family of genes, is a plausible asthma gene. The gene family includes $PDE4$, for which several inhibitors were found to have successfully suppressed inflammation; $PDE4A$, another newly reported asthma susceptibility gene; and $PDE5$ (Sildenafil), more popularly known as Viagra. This last is a treatment for erectile dysfunction through its effect of dilating blood vessels and was also used to develop a drug to treat exercise-induced asthma. Why then did our paper require documentation of replication in the original publication before acceptance by the journal?

The search for SNP associations using hundreds of thousands of SNPs has highlighted an old problem in epidemiology. Where a large number of observations are made, the chance of falsely identifying a positive association is high. If three types of antiepileptic drugs used by pregnant mothers, each with two dose levels, are examined for their association with 25 congenital malformations (not an uncommon study design), then 150 comparisons will be made and between 7 and 8 of them will be expected to meet the nominal level of statistical significance, by chance alone. How can chance findings be distinguished from real ones? Traditionally, identifying real associations has invoked claims of biological plausibility, often from animal studies but, as discussed elsewhere, little reliance can be placed on this. Epidemiologists are experts at mining the huge literature of in vitro and animal studies to find support for their study findings, whatever they might be. The most important validation of a research result is that it has been replicated in another study, preferably by a different research team. This follows the oldest tradition in science, that observations should be verifiable. Because of the virtual certainty of false positive results in the new hypothesis-free genomic research, journals are quite properly requesting a replication of findings, even in the original publication. Fortunately this does not always entail much additional work as published genetic databases may be rapidly scanned to check the strength of the new association of interest with a particular genetic variant.

It is not always clear what the level of replication should be. The gene-rather than SNP-level replication that we selected is one choice, but there are many more. It is known that gene function can be disturbed by variations in many possible SNPs. Also, how precisely should the disease classification (what is called the phenotype) be copied? If the disease type is not exactly the same between studies, then failure to replicate an association may be owed to each variant of the disease having a different set of causative factors. How important is it that the patients in the different studies are similar (not replicating a finding in a different ethnic group, for example, may simply reflect differences on other important factors, including culture and genetics), and how closely should the therapeutic intervention or suspected causative environmental agent vary (drugs demonstrate different properties even within the same drug class or at different doses of the same drug)? How many replications are required—two, half a dozen, or more? For replication to be meaningful, scientists have always demanded, if not exact then quite similar replication. Any variation in study design provides a loophole for explaining why a replication may not have been successful except for the most important reason: the initial observation was due to chance.

Simple replication has been surpassed by the concept of pooling and meta-analysis. Replication by itself is of little benefit unless all of the studies on the same topic are collected and formally examined, a process called "systematic reviewing." The number of replications is irrelevant; what matters is the quality ("validity" is the technical term used) of the replicated or pooled evidence. Rarely, one very large well-conducted randomized trial may be considered adequate evidence. The 10,000 patient CRASH trial of the steroid methylprednisolone used to treat head injury, described in chapter 5, is unlikely to be replicated given the compelling results that the steroid was harmful and the resources that would be needed to launch another very large trial. In contrast, the evidence that Vioxx (rofecoxib) increased risk of myocardial infarctions became compelling only after a dozen trials had been done and they were systematically reviewed and meta-analyzed as discussed in more detail below.[4] The science of systematic reviewing, which may or may not include a meta-analysis depending on the quality of the available data, is one of the great scientific breakthroughs in medicine and health care of the twentieth century.

Pooling Scientific Data

In his superb account of the origins of empirical medicine, focusing on its early history in Britain, Ulrich Tröhler documents the development of evidence-based and quantitative medicine arising from a foundation among the late eighteenth-century "arithmetic observationists and experimentalists." These pioneers in the use of statistics and probability for evaluating the success of medical therapies are exemplified by an Irish physician William Black, who in his text *An Arithmetical and Medical Analysis of the Diseases and Mortality of the Human Species* wrote somewhat poetically in 1789, "However it may be slighted as an heretical innovation, I would strenuously recommend Medical Arithmetick, as a guide and compass through the labyrinth of the therapeutic." These mathematical doctors were known for compiling death statistics, analyzing their case records, making comparisons of treated patients with "controls," and conducting experiments on the usefulness of therapies that are recognizable as the earliest, albeit primitive by modern standards, medical trials.[5]

Like many scientific revolutions, the use of mathematics in quantifying medical experience was slow to be adopted into widespread practice (indeed, there are isolated medical specialties that to this day appear to remain oblivious to the need for empirical investigation). Nonetheless, by the mid-nineteenth century academic medicine was more widely accepting of the value of medical statistics, and the early empiricists had sowed the first seeds of systematic reviewing: for example, comparing and contrasting the survival of patients seen by various doctors or being treated in different hospitals. One of the earliest published meta-analyses was performed in 1904 by Karl Pearson, professor of applied mathematics at University College, London, and one of the most eminent medical statisticians of his generation, whose work is also discussed in chapter 8. Pearson was investigating the rate of immunity and survival in cases of enteric fever according to whether the patient had an enteric fever inoculation from the experience in five different populations (four army regiments and several military hospitals involved in the South African war). Using a correlation statistic (a metric not favored by modern meta-analysts), Pearson was able to document considerable variation in the protective effect of the inoculation. What makes this a forerunner of modern meta-analysis is the recalculation of the effect of inoculation using the same statistic in each regiment's data, calculating an average correlation across all regiments, and the attention paid to "heterogeneity," that is, why the inoculation may have been successful in some regiments but less so in others. To explain the observed heterogeneity, Fisher invokes an early example of what is now called selection bias, in which the more cautious soldiers are the ones seeking inoculation and also avoiding exposure to fever, suggesting "a real correlation between immunity and caution." Fisher concludes that routine inoculation against enteric fever could not be justified, and he calls for an experiment where volunteers are registered but only "every second volunteer" is inoculated. Interestingly, this paper anticipates current recommendations that proposals for new clinical trials should include a meta-analysis of the existing evidence (although the quasi-randomization scheme proposed by Fisher would be frowned on).[6]

Possibly the first meta-analysis conducted in the United States was published in 1907 by Goldberger (whose work on pellagra was discussed extensively in chapter 1). In this study, Goldberger had turned his attention to the then urgent question of how typhoid carriers could be diagnosed using the presence of the typhoid bacillus in their urine. There were 44 study reports from which Goldberger selected 26 that had used a new serum agglutination test and had randomly selected patients for testing. From these studies, Goldberger extracted the data and recalculated a typical rate of 16 percent for the bacillus to be found in urine. While not a modern method for estimating the value of a diagnostic test (see chapter 7), this report showed the poor predictive value of a negative urine test.[7]

Archibald Leman (Archie) Cochrane (1909–1988) was a British physician who, after capture in Crete in 1941, found himself a prisoner of war and camp medical officer for four years, treating the other prisoners, often for tuberculosis. A prisoner of war camp was an environment with scarce resources and Cochrane realized that treating patients with limited supplies might more ethically be accomplished in a random fashion. After the war he worked at the British Medical Research Council's pneumoconiosis (a lung disease common in coal miners) research unit where, his obituary noted, he developed "an obsessional interest in reproducibility."[8] The work for which he is best known started in 1969 when he began promoting the increased use of randomized controlled trials to test treatments being used in another resource-scarce environment, the National Health Service. In

1972 he published his landmark book *Effectiveness and Efficiency: Random Reflections on Health Services*, which was highly influential in promoting randomized trials. Cochrane died without really knowing that he was a major pioneer in evidence-based medicine. He concluded his self-penned obituary: "He was a man with severe porphyria who smoked too much and was without the consolation of a wife, a religious belief, or a merit award — but he didn't do so badly."[9]

The long arm of Cochrane is perhaps reflected in the comments of President Barack Obama who in 2009 remarked, "If there's a blue pill and a red pill, and the blue pill is half the price of the red pill and works just as well, why not pay half the price for the thing that's going to make you well?" This was anticipated in the *Economist* magazine's 1972 review of *Effectiveness and Efficiency:* "Dr. Cochrane does not ask for more money for the health service. He establishes a strong case for saying that enough could be found

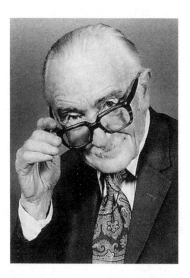

Figure 13.1. Archie Cochrane, 1909–1988. "It is surely a great criticism of our profession that we have not organized a critical summary by specialty or subspecialty, adapted periodically, of all relevant randomized controlled trials." Archie Cochrane, 1979. Courtesy Sir Iain Chalmers, James Lind Library.

to reduce the inequality between its curing branch and its caring one . . . if effective therapy were deployed to the right people, in the right place at the right time."

Archie Cochrane's mission was taken up by another British obstetrician and scientist, Iain Chalmers, whose international and long-lasting influence on medical and public health research started in the late 1970s when he founded the United Kingdom's National Perinatal Epidemiology Unit. Chalmers took to heart Cochrane's admonition "it is surely a great criticism of our profession that we have not organized a critical summary by specialty or subspecialty, adapted periodically, of all relevant randomized controlled trials," and he started to compile a database of all the clinical trials he could locate in obstetrics and neonatology.[10]

This work resulted in the Oxford Database of Perinatal Trials (ODPT), edited by Iain Chalmers and published by Oxford University Press in 1988 as a series of floppy discs. This monumental achievement represented the first compilation of randomized trials in any medical or any other kind of professional specialty. With computer access to the world's scientific literature now freely available, and with word indexing fine-tuned to make bibliographic searching relatively easy, it is difficult to appreciate the effort that was once needed to sieve through the literature to uncover randomized trials in the medical literature. In the winter of 1986–1987, personally signed letters from Chalmers were sent to more than 42,000 obstetricians and pediatricians seeking information about unpublished, ongoing, or planned trials, but the returns did not produce many unpublished trials. Only 18 trials were identified that had been completed more than two years before the survey and so might have been expected to have been published.[11]

In a ten-year period, over 3,000 randomized or quasi-randomized trials of interventions used during pregnancy or within 28 days of delivery, published since 1948, were identified for inclusion in ODPT. Also included were trial overviews and meta-analyses, the trial database, and editorial commentary on each overview.[12]

The concept for ODPT and its software was the prototype for what would become the Cochrane Collaboration, about which more later, but the immediate spin-off was two textbooks that represented the first attempt to provide the highest-quality evidence from randomized controlled trials for the most important interventions used in a medical specialty. The first, published in 1989, was *Effective Care in Pregnancy and Childbirth*, edited by Iain Chalmers, Murray Enkin, and Marc Keirse, followed in 1992 by *Effective Care of the Newborn Infant*, edited by John Sinclair and Michael Bracken.[13] These books were perceived at the time to be novel and a breakthrough in how evidence should be used to inform medical treatments. Each volume collated the evidence from ODPT and recruited specialists in each of the areas of therapy being reviewed to write chapters based on the trial evidence. Within the next decade, this model for systematically reviewing evidence was followed in virtually every other medical, and many nonmedical, specialties, with dozens of books been written using "evidence-based" strategies and systematic reviews to examine medical interventions.

In 1992, with support from the Research and Development Programme of the British National Health Service, Iain Chalmers led the establishment of "a Cochrane Centre," based in Oxford, to promote the adoption of similar strategies across all of health care. In 1993, the center convened a meeting at which the international Cochrane Collaboration was inaugurated.[14] Not surprisingly, given its origins, the first review groups were in pregnancy and

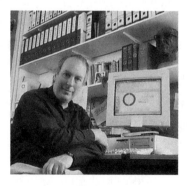

Figure 13.2. Sir Iain Chalmers, circa 2000. Sir Iain Chalmers, the founder of the Cochrane Collaboration with, on the lower shelf, ECPC, ECNI, ODPT, and a bust of Archie Cochrane. On the screen is the first edition of the Cochrane Library.

childbirth, subfertility, and neonatology, and they were based on the edito-rial and writing teams from the two "Effective Care" books. Also in 1993, ODPT was reissued as the Cochrane Pregnancy and Childbirth Database, which became the formal pilot for the Cochrane Library.[15]

In 2011, the Cochrane Collaboration had over 28,000 contributors in 100 countries organized into 52 review groups covering every aspect of health care and public health, and 13 Cochrane centers around the world provid-ing infrastructure and training support. In addition, there were 13 Cochrane methods groups responsible for developing the methodology to improve the science of systematic reviewing and meta-analysis, and 15 Cochrane field groups covering crosscutting topics such as child health. Over 2,000 jour-nals have been hand searched to identify reports of randomized trials, and over 650,000 trials had been registered in the Cochrane trials database.

The review groups are the heart of the collaboration as this is where the reviews are organized, prepared, and edited before entering the Cochrane Library. By 2012, over 5,000 reports of systematic reviews were in the Co-chrane Library, almost all based on evidence from randomized trials, and more than 2,000 protocols for reviews were registered, representing areas where reviews are currently being prepared. The Cochrane Collaboration is widely recognized today as being the single best source for high-quality systematic reviews in medicine and health care, and in 2011 the Cochrane Collaboration was awarded a seat at the World Health Organization's World Health Assembly being described by Marie-Paule Kieny, assistant director general of WHO, as "an international benchmark for the independent as-sessment and assimilation of scientific evidence."

The success of the Cochrane Collaboration has spawned several re-lated organizations with an interest in scientifically synthesizing research. The Campbell Collaboration was named after the eminent social science methodologist Donald T. Campbell (1916–1996), who recommended that experimental methods be used to evaluate government and federal agency social programs. It prepares systematic reviews in political science, crime and justice, social welfare, and education. The Human Genome Epide-miology Network (HuGENet), supported by the United States Centers for Disease Control, prepares systematic reviews of associations between ge-

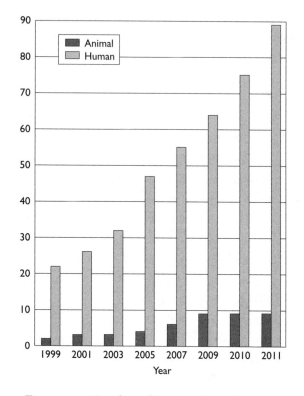

Figure 13.3. Number of meta-analyses for every
10,000 publications in PubMed, 1999–2011.

netic variations and disease, and other groups are organizing to conduct
systematic reviews of animal studies and toxicology. Outside of these collaborations, systematic reviewing and meta-analysis has grown rapidly over
the last decade throughout the medical literature, as shown by data from the
United States National Library of Medicine's database, MEDLINE.

Figure 13.3 shows the increase in the annual number of meta-analyses
published in MEDLINE over the last 10 years as a proportion of the total number of publications being published annually. In 1999, for human
studies, there were just over 20 meta-analyses for every 10,000 publications,
annually, which has quadrupled in the last decade to more than 80 (in ab-

solute numbers, from about 700 annually to more than 4,000). The number of animal study meta-analyses is much smaller and seems to have reached a plateau in recent years.

Systematic Reviews and Meta-Analysis

A systematic review, just as all scientific research, requires a specific hypothesis which is called a focused question and which typically has four parts: (1) identify a specific group of patients or the public to be studied, (2) describe a specific intervention, (3) define a comparison to an alternative intervention, including doing nothing, and (4) examine whether there is an observable effect on a specific set of health outcomes. The question is structured slightly differently for other types of research, for example, a screening or diagnosis question would be: given the pretest probability of disease and a test result, what is the posttest probability of disease? An example of a focused intervention question is: among children with mite-sensitive asthma, do house dust mite control measures (using chemical or physical means), compared with placebo control or no control measures, reduce asthma symptoms?

To examine what the relevant literature on a research question demonstrates, a comprehensive literature search must be conducted. There are some 15,000 medical journals publishing well over a million articles annually, and unless the search is properly focused, far too many articles will be obtained for detailed scrutiny. On the other hand, a narrower search may miss important papers. Therefore, properly constructed searches are required. An entire science in literature searching has evolved over the last twenty years to help with this. Another choice that must be made is the study design; our example is a "treatment" question (here the home environment is being manipulated to reduce mites), and the design to test it reliably is the randomized controlled trial. Indeed, many investigators consider any other type of design for "treatment" studies to be so inferior that they should be ignored. The search for studies is then limited to trials that had used an unbiased treatment allocation. If no eligible trials are found from the literature search, the conclusion of the review may be that no reliable evidence exists to assess the effects of the intervention, a result which should prompt further, higher-quality research.

The next question, at the literature searching stage of the systematic review, is whether to include all languages. Language bias, the preference for sending studies with positive results to the most high-profile journals (which typically publish in English), is well documented, and so not using any language limitation is recommended. Whether or not to include abstracts and other non-peer-reviewed papers is also debated. Next, to match the focused question, the population under study must be specified, the treatments and comparison groups detailed, and the outcomes of interest described in detail. Usually one to three primary outcomes, which are the conditions most likely to be affected by the intervention, are defined. In our example, lung volume measured by peak flow, reported asthma symptoms, or use of asthma medication might all be examined. The secondary outcomes are of related importance and in this example may include hospitalizations for asthma.

When the search has produced studies that appear to be relevant to the review question, each report is examined in detail to assess the methodological rigor with which the research was conducted. Even if studies of treatments are restricted to randomized controlled trials, there is variability in how well the trials were conducted and whether bias was well controlled. For each trial there are four principal biases that are of concern, addressed by four questions:

> *Was an unbiased allocation schedule adequately concealed?* If the allocation schedule (typically called the randomization schedule) was not concealed, the entry of patients into the trial may have been biased as a doctor may decide to exclude a patient even if she only *thinks* the randomized treatment is going to be, say, placebo. The operative word is "thinks" because even though the treatments are hidden, systematically withdrawing patients after randomization may introduce bias into the study.
>
> *Were the interventions being provided adequately masked?* If the randomized intervention therapies are not masked, difficul-

ties arise when other ways of managing the patient are altered to "compensate" for what is being given, or not given, in the trial. No longer will the patients in the trial comparison groups be similar on every characteristic except the randomized treatments they received, which seriously undermines interpretation of the trial.

Was the follow-up reasonably complete? If the number of patients followed up is not high, the results from those who are followed may differ from those who drop out to a degree that the observed results may be invalid. Most trials aim for at least a 95 percent follow-up rate.

Was the assessment of the outcome masked? If the people assessing the trial outcome are aware of which treatment the patient received, their reporting of the clinical outcome may be biased. If death is the outcome, it is not always easy to attribute death to a specific cause, and this may be biased by knowledge of therapy. Even if all-cause mortality is assessed, the search for information to confirm the death may vary with knowledge of which treatment was received.

Once the validity of each trial has been assessed, the systematic reviewer will abstract the relevant data from the trial and may include it in a meta-analysis. The principal concerns at this stage involve the comparability of the data and whether they are sufficiently similar to provide reliable estimates of efficacy and risk. Lack of similarity may be owed to differences in the interventions used in different studies (for mite remediation: a different type of air filter, various mattress covers, a regimen for cleaning the home), variations in the entry criteria for patients in the trials (age or gender differences, variations in the clinical criteria of the disease being studied), and using different measures to assess the outcome (variation in asthma severity assessment scales, different assays, and when the outcome was measured after treatment: 4 weeks, 6 months, a year). Some of these differences may have been anticipated in the review protocol for examination in subgroup comparisons, but others may emerge only later. If a meta-analysis seems justified after reviewing the quality of the data, this is done using standard statistical methods. However, systematic reviews that cannot conduct a meta-analysis still perform the useful function of describing an area of clinical or public health practice that is not based on high-quality evidence.

In the house dust mite control example, a Cochrane review found 54 randomized trials — 36 using physical interventions (typically, mattress coverings), 10 chemical approaches, and 8 mixing both strategies. The trials were of generally poor quality, and none of the interventions had any detectable effect on peak flow measured in the morning, asthma symptom scores, or asthma medication use.[16]

Meta-analyses of high-quality randomized trials by themselves may be taken as evidence that a causal relationship has been established: a therapy does cause improvement, or it does cause harm. However, lack of effectiveness or lack of harm (that is, safety) is not formally proven by a null result. Trials are testing the null hypothesis, no difference in efficacy or harm between the experimental and control groups, and the null hypothesis can only be formally rejected, it cannot be accepted (chapter 8). Nonetheless, lack of efficacy and safety are assumed as a practical matter and guide medical and public health practice accordingly.

Vioxx

We will use Vioxx as an example of how the results from several randomized trials can provide reliable evidence as to causality. Vioxx (rofecoxib) is a nonsteroidal anti-inflammatory drug and a member of the COX-2 inhibitor drugs that were developed to provide pain relief from osteoarthritis with the added benefit of not increasing the risk of stomach ulceration. A Cochrane review of 26 randomized trials including over 21,000 people showed quite clearly that Vioxx is an effective pain reliever compared to placebo (29 percent of patients reported less pain on placebo, 53 percent on Vioxx), but there was mixed evidence for risk of stomach ulceration.[17] The controversial problem for Vioxx arose with evidence that it was increasing the risk of heart attacks, especially in people already at increased risk. This evidence came from the VIGOR trial conducted by the manufacturer, Merck Pharmaceuticals. It indicated a fourfold increased risk of heart attack in the Vioxx users compared with patients taking another nonsteroidal anti-inflammatory drug, Naproxen, the rates being 4 per 1,000 compared with 1 per 1,000. Given the rarity of these events, and the knowledge that this difference is readily achieved by chance, one needs to turn to a meta-analysis and one was available. What does it show? Peter Jüni and colleagues from Switzerland provided a meta-analysis that was published in the *Lancet* in 2004; figure 13.4 shows the essential data. Sixteen trials addressed the question of

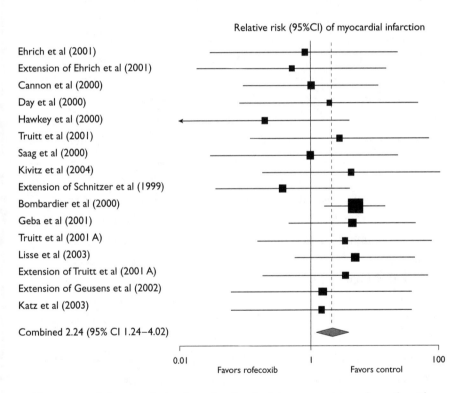

Figure 13.4. Meta-analysis of randomized trials comparing rofecoxib with control. Reprinted from *The Lancet:* Jüni P, Nartey L, Reichenbach S, Sterchi R, Dieppe PA, Egger M. Risk of cardiovascular events and rofecoxib: cumulative meta-analysis. *Lancet.* 2004;364(9450):2021–2029. Copyright 2004, with permission from Elsevier.

heart attack after Vioxx versus control, and the increased risk was 124 percent (RR = 2.24 95%CI 1.24, 4.02), which was statistically significant.

How was the meta-analysis result calculated? The number of heart attacks experienced by patients in each treatment group is reported for each trial and the respective relative risk calculated (chapter 8 describes the calculation). The influence of each trial is then weighted by the overall effect that each trial has on the summary statistic calculated by the meta-analysis. Those trials having the largest number of heart attacks contribute the most weight; the size of the black box in the figure reflects the weight. Figure 13.4 shows that only one of the sixteen trials (Bombardier et al.) was large enough to demonstrate a statistically significant result by itself; all the others were imprecise, with four suggesting a protective effect. Jüni and colleagues conducted additional statistical analyses to confirm that their results were not influenced by the Vioxx dose, if the control group received placebo or another active drug, and how long the trial lasted. Because this meta-analysis is based on randomized trials, it provides quite powerful evidence that there is at least a doubling of cardiovascular risk in patients using Vioxx. By itself, however, the analysis does not address if there is a particular type of patient who is at increased risk, what the risk benefit is for reducing pain, or protecting against gastric ulceration all of which requires additional data. Importantly, this type of analysis addresses general causation and does not provide direct evidence that a heart attack in any individual patient was caused by using Vioxx. In a related editorial, the *Lancet* editors report that the United States FDA estimated that 27,000 excess cases of acute myocardial infarction and sudden cardiac death had resulted from Vioxx use between 1999 and 2003, a reflection of its widespread use, which may have included 80 million persons worldwide.[18]

In contrast to trial-based meta-analyses, those using observational studies can be quite misleading. An example was shown in chapter 6 of the meta-analysis of case-control studies of prior induced abortion that spuriously suggested an increased risk of breast cancer. The biases in observational data are amplified in meta-analysis, giving more precision to an incorrect risk estimate. This is particularly so in case-control studies, and many scientists are of the view that case-control studies should never be meta-analyzed. Meta-analyses of *prospective* observational studies may have a role to play, especially when the exposures and conditions being studied are so rare that any individual study, however large, is unlikely to produce a reliable result. An example of this occurred when trying to review the literature concerning the risk of rare birth defects after oral contraceptive exposure. Specific birth defects occur at a rate of only one or two per thousand births, and oral contraception is a rare exposure, not least because it is so successful at preventing pregnancy. Nonetheless, some pregnancies follow soon after oral contraceptive use and others occur as a "breakthrough" pregnancy during use. These are the pregnancies of interest. The results of a meta-analysis are shown in figure 13.5.

Even in a very large study of over 50,000 participants, the estimate of risk for limb reduction malformation was imprecise, with very wide confidence intervals, but when the studies are combined, with over 90,000 study respondents in total, a statistically reasonably robust estimate is obtained: in this example, that there is no increased risk of a baby having a limb reduction malformation after exposure from oral contraceptives.[19] Being able to improve the precision of risk estimates is one of the unique strengths of meta-analysis.

Cumulative Meta-Analysis

It is often important to discover at what point in time a treatment may be judged, with reasonable certainty, to be effective or, alternatively, has been shown to be unsafe. A procedure called cumulative meta-analysis, which ranks the studies in chronological order and calculates the estimate of risk each time a study is added to the accumulating evidence, is useful for this. An example is shown in figure 13.6 from the same Vioxx trials shown in a conventional meta-analysis in figure 13.4. This analysis shows that by the year 2001 there was compelling evidence for an increased risk of heart attack with Vioxx, that is, three years before it was withdrawn from the market in September of 2004 (figure 13.6).

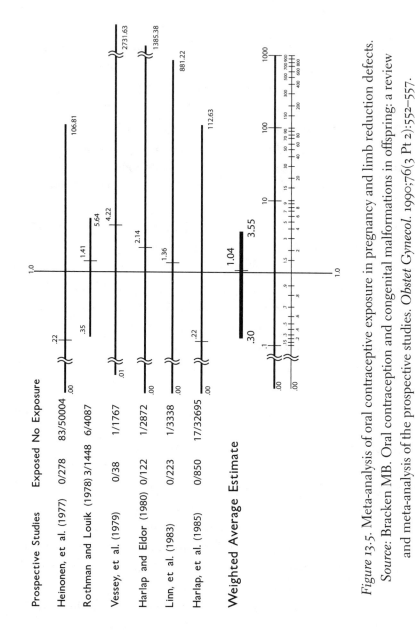

Figure 13.5. Meta-analysis of oral contraceptive exposure in pregnancy and limb reduction defects. *Source:* Bracken MB. Oral contraception and congenital malformations in offspring: a review and meta-analysis of the prospective studies. *Obstet Gynecol.* 1990;76(3 Pt 2):552–557.

Year	Patients	Events	p
1997	523	1	0.916
1998	615	2	0.736
	1,399	5	0.828
	2,208	6	0.996
	2,983	8	0.649
	3,324	9	0.866
1999	4,017	12	0.879
	5,059	13	0.881
2000	5,193	16	0.855
	13,269	40	0.070
	14,247	44	0.034
	15,156	46	0.025
	20,742	52	0.010
	20,742	58	0.007
2001	20,742	63	0.007
	21,432	64	0.007

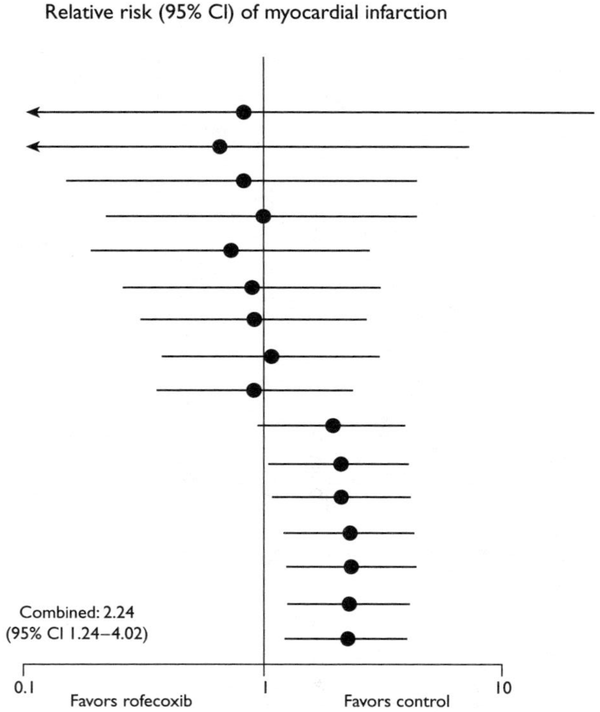

Relative risk (95% CI) of myocardial infarction

Combined: 2.24
(95% CI 1.24–4.02)

Favors rofecoxib   Favors control

Figure 13.6. Cumulative meta-analysis of the risk for myocardial infarction associated with *Vioxx.* Reprinted from the *Lancet*: Jüni P, Nartey L, Reichenbach S, Sterchi R, Dieppe PA, Egger M. Risk of cardiovascular events and rofecoxib: cumulative meta-analysis. *Lancet.* 2004;364(9450):2021–2029. Copyright 2004, with permission from Elsevier. The Merck Pharmaceutical Company responded to the Jüni paper, claiming it had not included all the relevant trials.

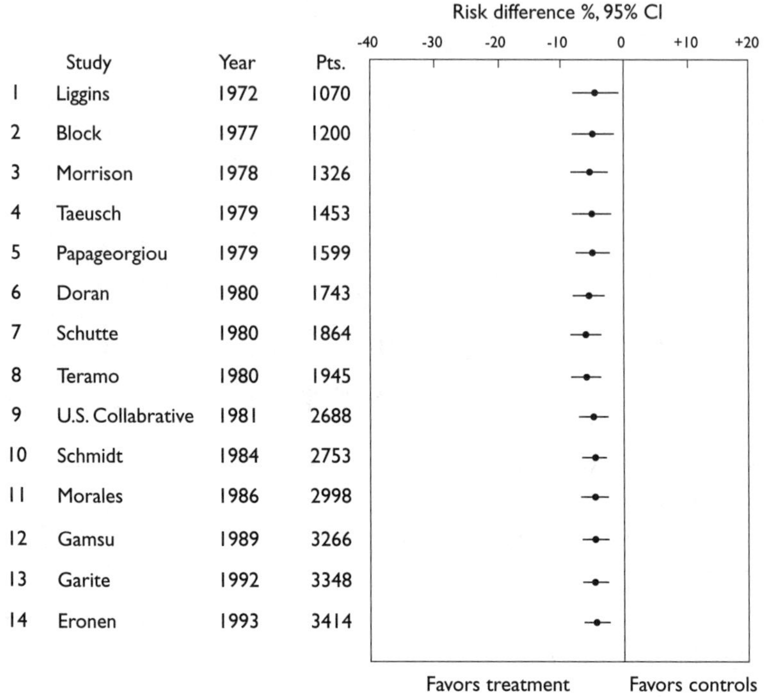

	Study	Year	Pts.	Risk difference %, 95% CI
1	Liggins	1972	1070	
2	Block	1977	1200	
3	Morrison	1978	1326	
4	Taeusch	1979	1453	
5	Papageorgiou	1979	1599	
6	Doran	1980	1743	
7	Schutte	1980	1864	
8	Teramo	1980	1945	
9	U.S. Collabrative	1981	2688	
10	Schmidt	1984	2753	
11	Morales	1986	2998	
12	Gamsu	1989	3266	
13	Garite	1992	3348	
14	Eronen	1993	3414	

Favors treatment   Favors controls

Figure 13.7. Cumulative meta-analysis of the effect of antenatal steroids given to mothers in preterm labor on risk of death of the newborn. Reprinted from: Sinclair JC. Meta-analysis of randomized controlled trials of antenatal corticosteroid for the prevention of respiratory distress syndrome: discussion. *Am J Obstet Gynecol.* 1995;173(1): 335–344. Copyright 1995, with permission from Elsevier.

Cumulative meta-analysis is also useful for demonstrating the unnecessary continuation of experiments and trials after benefit has been convincingly documented. An example from the animal studies of tPA and stroke was shown in chapter 11. Figure 13.7 shows an example from human trials in neonatology. In 1972, Graham Liggins and Ross Howie, an obstetrician and a pediatrician from Auckland, New Zealand, followed up on many studies their team had conducted on the most popular newborn animal model in their country, lambs, to assess whether antenatal steroids given to 1,070 mothers in preterm labor would reduce the problems associated with pre-term birth, which were frequently fatal conditions. Their trial showed a significant reduction in neonatal mortality with an absolute reduction in risk of 4.5 percent; that is, for every 22 mothers treated, 1 newborn's life would be saved, certainly a worthwhile intervention. After a report of the first trial was published there were 13 more trials, all much smaller in size, suggesting either a protective or no effect. When the data for all these trials were eventually analyzed in a systematic review and meta-analysis, this showed that the treatment resulted in a very important reduction in neonatal morbidity and death.[20]

The data in figure 13.7 was put together retrospectively in 1995 by an eminent neonatologist John C. Sinclair and showed that had a contemporary cumulative analysis been maintained of the evidence as it was being reported over the previous two decades, it would have been observed that the treatment always showed statistically significant protection; as more trials were published, the estimate of reduced risk didn't change, it simply was estimated with more confidence. Trials started after 1980 seem to have been redundant, and the newborns of mothers given placebo in them were placed at unnecessary risk.[21]

The importance of electronic publishing as a way of updating evidence with the results of every new trial was noted in the mid 1980s,[22] inaugurated with the release of the Oxford Database of Perinatal Trials,[23] and applied retrospectively and named cumulative meta-analysis in 1992.[24] The antenatal steroid analysis also points to a feature of conducting multiple trials on the same topic, if one trial has been published, there is little point conducting another one that is smaller. For new evidence to have any chance of influencing the current risk estimate, subsequent trials must be larger and should improve on any design problems with the first trial, none of which was evident in the later antenatal steroids trials.

Individual Patient Data Meta-Analyses

The importance of obtaining large-scale randomized evidence for causal associations was discussed in the context of large simple trials (chapter 5), and a second way of finding these data is described here. It is called "individual patient data meta-analysis" (IPDMA) and has been pioneered by researchers in Cambridge, Oxford, and London, in particular. In this procedure, raw data from individual randomized trials contributing to a topic are combined in a single computer repository where they can be cleaned, checked, and reanalyzed. The risk estimates are then recalculated for each trial and analyzed as in a traditional meta-analysis, described above. The advantages are manifold: additional follow-up data can be obtained and "time to event" analysis is made possible, which in cancer trials is one of the principal outcomes, and this, although perhaps assessed differently in the individual trials, can now be unified. Event-free survival is another common outcome, but the definition of what is an event may also vary among different trials and this can be standardized by IPDMA. Also, subgroups may have been defined in different ways, and analyses of subgroups, while always suspect, may be undertaken with caution in an IPDMA which allows for more robust analysis of rare outcomes.[25]

The IPDMA strategy has been called the "gold standard" of meta-analysis and has led to several important consortia being developed including the Early Breast Cancer Trialists' Collaborative Group, which showed the benefit of Tamoxifen therapy continuing as long as 10 years after treatment as well as the benefit to long-term survival of ovarian ablation in women under age 50 with breast cancer.[26] A more recent IPDMA was able to provide clear clinical guidance on the effectiveness of single versus double embryo transfer from fresh IVF cycles, using data from eight trials involving 1,367 women. Pooling data allowed several aspects of the transfer procedure to be examined that no single trial could have done. A live birth occurred 27 percent of the time after single embryo transfer and 42 percent of the time after double; however, a singleton pregnancy was almost five time more likely after single embryo transfer and two successive single embryo transfers resulted in a singleton *birth* 38 percent of the time, not substantially different from the double embryo transfer rate and without the risk associated with having a twin birth.[27]

"This toothpaste has been recommended by more dentists!" used to be the typical basis for claims of superior effectiveness. Despite increased regulation and a greatly improved research methodology for evaluating evidence of claims made for medical therapies, in many respects the public continues to be deluged with unproven recommendations and advice. "Clinically proven" is still touted, but the reference is usually not to a well-conducted systematic review of randomized trial evidence but to a small marketing-driven piece of work falling far short of rigorous scientific standards. Data replication remains essential to validate the results of individual studies, but, as we have seen, data pooling and meta-analysis go far beyond mere replication. They can now provide additional evidence that individual studies are unable to produce, and they have become a vital tool in the search for causation.

FOURTEEN

Bias in Publication and Reporting

The great tragedy of science is the slaying of a
beautiful hypothesis by an ugly fact.
—*Thomas Henry Huxley, 1870*

Don't confuse hypothesis and theory. The former is a
possible explanation; the latter, the correct one. The
establishment of theory is the very purpose of science.
—*Martin H. Fischer*

Traditionally, scientific knowledge has been obtained by developing hypotheses that can be tested in a study or experiment designed to produce data that will either support or refute it. As Huxley satirically put it in his presidential address to the British Association for the Advancement of Science, science is littered with beautiful but failed hypotheses. In the modern medical sciences, we are less reliant on the results of a single study, preferring to see replication in several of them and their confirmation within the framework of a systematic review and meta-analysis. Nonetheless, the scientific paradigm of hypothesis testing prevails: the hypothesis is typically laid out in a study protocol to describe exactly what is being tested and the precise outcome expected. It is not easy for scientists to discard what often becomes a favored and long-held hypothesis. Konrad Lorenz, the influential behavioral zoologist, advised: "It is a good morning exercise for a research scientist to discard a pet hypothesis every day before breakfast. It keeps him young."

In this chapter, we discuss situations where the hypothesis testing construct is deliberately violated by not publishing studies that fail to support a preferred hypothesis, by reporting them in a manner that conceals what the actual hypothesis was, or, even worse, by misrepresenting the original hypothesis. Hypotheses are not discarded but rather are transmuted during publication to something entirely different, and in so doing, the safety of the public is severely jeopardized.

Some years ago I was asked by a very large pharmaceutical company to review the evidence supporting a glossy advertising campaign being run in the leading medical journals touting the claim by another equally large company that its antihypertensive drug was superior to that of my client's. Reference was made in the advertisement to a small, randomized trial of only 32 subjects, which documented a marginal clinical improvement in the other company's product compared with my client's drug. The trial was unimpressive, clearly subject to being wrong, and had any of the prescribing doctors to whom the expensive advertising was aimed bothered to look up the citation, they assuredly would not have been impressed. During the pretrial depositions, it was discovered that a second (equally unimpressive) trial of similar size had been conducted and was found residing in a file drawer with no plans to publish. Perhaps not surprisingly, this trial showed an equally modest improvement, but this time the benefit was to the patients treated with my client's drug. A simple meta-analysis combining data from the two trials showed absolutely no difference in the clinical effectiveness of the two antihypertensive drugs. The other company's drug was not superior to that of my client's. The Food and Drug Administration (FDA), which has regulatory control over pharmaceutical company advertising, was extremely annoyed, and the lawsuit between the companies was quickly settled.

What had been observed in the above anecdote is a classic (and literal) example of what is called "file drawer bias"; this is the inclination of investigators (academic as well as corporate) to write up and submit for publication those results that favor their employer's product, their long-held hypotheses, or their perceived chances of achieving tenure. Not only would the doctors examining the citation to the antihypertensive medication not have been impressed with the paper that was cited, they would have had no way of knowing that another trial, producing the opposite result, had been conducted. File drawer bias is one aspect of a larger set of problems in reporting studies: "publication bias." This is a particularly pernicious source of bias when investigators are conducting a meta-analysis that seeks to summarize the totality of evidence on any particular topic. If the literature is biased by selective publication of positive results, then conclusions drawn about the effectiveness of therapies will be wrong. This bias can have life-threatening consequences.

Hexamethonium is a blood pressure medication that was used in a study funded by Johns Hopkins University and the National Institutes of Health to try and understand how asthma symptoms developed. The study had to be suspended when one of its participants, a previously healthy 24-year-old woman, died of lung collapse soon after taking the medication. The investigation committee, established by Johns Hopkins to look into the death, examined how thorough a literature search was conducted by the investigator to identify potential drug complications before he submitted his research protocol to the ethics review committee. It turned out, using a standard PubMed search and consulting current textbooks, that some key studies had been missed. The ethics committee, after the research volunteer's death, conducted a search of several bibliographic databases and in reviewing material from the 1950s found earlier work suggesting pulmonary side effects from hexamethonium. In a letter to the NIH oversight office, a university dean wrote, "The committee was divided on the issue of what constitutes a sufficient search of the literature in support of a human subjects research application."[1] Even in 2011, a search using the Johns Hopkins investigator's name and hexamethonium produced no results in PubMed, but it found eleven using Google Scholar, a reflection of the inadequacy of relying solely on a PubMed search.[2] One can only speculate that perhaps it is due to legal advice that no complete report of this failed experiment can be found in the literature. Hopefully, no one in the future will attempt to replicate this failed experiment, but if they do, inadequate reporting of the first study can only increase the chance of repeated disaster.

The proclivity for pharmaceutical companies to publish only the results of studies that favor their products was formally investigated by a group of scientists interested in antidepressant drugs. Using an innovative strategy, they obtained the results of trials submitted by pharmaceutical companies for review to the FDA to seek licensing approval. Some of the information was obtained under the US Freedom of Information Act and is unlikely to have otherwise seen the light of day. The results of the trials in the FDA files were then compared to published reports in the medical literature. In all, 74 FDA-registered studies were located concerning 12 antidepressant agents and 12,564 patients. Whether or not the drug was found to be efficacious in treating depression, and the size of the benefit, was judged using the FDA's own determination during the regulatory process.

The results were striking: 38 trials met the criterion for a positive effect and 37 were published. In contrast, of the 36 trials considered negative or questionable by the FDA, only 3 were subsequently published. In short, the positive studies were 12 times more likely to be published than the negative ones. The net effect of this was that the published literature suggested 94 percent of the trials were positive but the FDA analysis indicated only 51 percent as being positive. Even among the published trials found to be positive by the FDA, the published effect size was on average 32 percent greater in the published reports than obtained in the FDA review. Were the unpublished studies inferior in some respect that might explain their lack of publication? The review authors could find no evidence for this: the studies were of similar size, and all the protocols had been written to meet international guidelines for drug efficacy studies. Finally, it was noted that this, quite depressing, bias in publication occurred among all the drugs studied and all the studied pharmaceutical companies.[3]

It has been estimated that some 25 to 50 percent of all studies are never published; in one project Kay Dickersin, one of the leading investigators into publication bias, followed up on studies whose protocols were submitted to ethics committees for review at several institutions and found that 8 to 14 years later 7 to 45 percent remained unpublished. The fewest unpublished trials were among the large NIH-sponsored clinical trials. When investigators were asked why their results were unpublished, the most frequently cited reason was that the results were "uninteresting."[4] In another study asking scientists why they delayed publication of their results for more than six months, the most frequent replies were to allow time for patent application, because of the proprietary or financial value of results, or to preserve the investigators' scientific lead, but 28 percent admitted it was intended to delay dissemination of undesired results.[5]

It is known that those studies that are published tend to favor what are called "positive" results; that is, results that find a definite answer to the research question, usually an increased risk for a suspected environmental exposure or a benefit for therapeutic research. Publication bias, therefore, is defined as the tendency toward the preparation, submission, and publication of research findings, based on the nature and direction of the results. As the definition indicates, it occurs across the publication spectrum: from the investigators' eagerness or not to write up a study report, deciding to which journal to submit it, and to the editor's willingness to accept the paper for publication. It has been found that statistically significant published study results are reported more frequently in journals with higher-impact factors (that is, their articles are cited by more researchers). Similarly, more statistically significant results are also found in higher-impact journals.[6]

John Ioannidis reported that all but a few "positive" trials were submitted for publication as late as two and a half years after completion but as many as one-fifth of negative trials remained unsubmitted even five years after completion. After submission, the median time for a positive trial to publication was just under one year but for a negative trial it was a few months longer.[7] Stern and Simes examined publication delay in a variety of quantitative studies from the time they were submitted for ethics committee approval to publication. Studies reporting statistically significant results fared best: only 1.4 percent remained unpublished after 10 years compared with 13.5 percent of the statistically nonsignificant studies.[8]

It is also known that only a small proportion of citations recovered by electronic searching of the major literature databases are relevant for the inquiry at hand. Clinical trials are particularly difficult to find; only about half of all relevant trials are successfully retrieved in a typical search on

the largest database, MEDLINE.[9] This is largely due to incomplete indexing of RCTs so that searching for text words (which is usually restricted
to the abstract) can fail to detect a randomized study. This limitation has
forced the Cochrane Collaboration, described earlier as the leading organization that maintains a register of reports of clinical trials, to hand search
hundreds of journals so that more reports of clinical trials can be correctly
identified.

Another aspect of publication bias concerns the language in which a paper has been written. Research has shown that non-English-language papers
are of similar quality to those written in English; however, they are more
likely to have statistically nonsignificant results. This is exemplified by a
hypothetical trial result at Stockholm University—if the results are positive
and considered to be important the paper is likely sent to one of the four
most widely read general clinical journals (the *Lancet, BMJ* [formerly *British Medical Journal*], *New England Journal of Medicine,* and *JAMA [Journal
of the American Medical Association]*), all of which publish in English. If
the results are considered null and perhaps not very interesting, they may be
more likely to be submitted to a Swedish journal publishing in that language.
Not only are non-English-speaking journals less accessible on MEDLINE
and other large bibliographic research databases, searches on MEDLINE
are often restricted to the English-language journals. Imagine how many
important studies of acupuncture would be missed if those in non-English
languages were to be excluded from a literature search.

Other pertinent research reports may be found in what is called the gray
literature. These are internal company or foundation reports, industry files,
and academic dissertations. Some research reports are known only because
of personal knowledge. Abstracts of presentations at scientific meetings are
another source of information although care in interpreting them is warranted: many investigators have to produce an abstract to be able to attend
conferences, but the abstract may represent incomplete, premature, or biased results that will not be confirmed when the study is finally completed.

We started this chapter with examples whereby unfavorable trial results
were being withheld, and an incomplete literature search had fatal consequences for a research volunteer. Publication bias is important for more

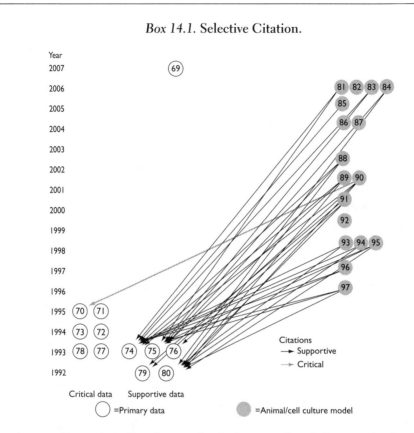

Box 14.1. Selective Citation.

Year

Citations
→ Supportive
→ Critical

Critical data   Supportive data

○ =Primary data   ● =Animal/cell culture model

In a revealing analysis, Greenberg used a citation network analysis to examine how individual papers published over a 15-year period were being cited. His example concerned a
theory that a particular amyloid protein is present in muscle, the details of which need not
concern us here. He found that the early studies supporting the theory were disproportionately cited over studies reporting nonsupportive data; even the same research group failed
to cite their previous papers if they did not support later results in favor of the theory. In
one analysis, there were 6 initial papers critical of the theory and 5 supportive, but among
17 subsequent publications, 16 failed to refer to any of the earlier critical studies. Grant
applications on the same topic were especially prone to citation bias; 6 of the 9 applications analyzed failed to mention any of the 6 critical papers, and 3 applications cited only
1 critical paper each. In contrast, 4 of the 5 supportive references were cited by all the
applications.

Other work shows what was called the "conversion of hypothesis to fact through citation alone" phenomenon; that is, publications misrepresent the earlier papers they cite as
having reported a finding as a fact when it was really presented only as a hypothesis.*

*Adapted by permission from BMJ Publishing Group Limited. (How citation distortions create un-
founded authority: analysis of a citation network, Greenberg SA, 339:b2680, Copyright 2009.)

prosaic reasons. First, we rely on the published literature to represent the true nature of current knowledge. Scientific progress is substantially hindered if the complete picture of what is currently known is perverted; this will lead to unnecessary replication and possible delay in making new therapeutic advances. Science, even at its best, goes through many twists and turns, false leads, and dead ends; it does not need the added complication of a misleading representation of the extant literature. Second, systematic reviews of the published literature are the source for clinical guidelines and policy statements. If the literature being used is a biased and incomplete picture of the full state of knowledge, the guidelines and policy may be wrong, resulting in needless risk and hazard for individual patients and the public.

One example of this concerns pregnant women with Group B streptococcal infections. Several years ago, a Centers for Disease Control guideline committee promulgated a recommendation that all women about to deliver a baby be tested for Group B strep and those testing positive (about 20 percent of the population) be given antibiotics for at least four hours before delivery. If a four-hour course could not be given, typically because the woman went into labor and delivered, it was recommended that the newborn have blood cultures drawn and be placed under observation, often in the newborn intensive care unit (NICU) or other observation area. This guideline resulted in tens of thousands of babies being separated from their mothers immediately after birth and placed in a NICU.

My colleague Jessica Illuzzi, a young academic obstetrician, took the bold step of questioning this guideline by reexamining the guideline committee's work. She found no evidence that it had conducted a systematic review of the relevant literature to inform its deliberations, and so Jessica did one herself: it provided no evidence to support the four-hour course of antibiotics.[10] In other work, she found that antibiotic levels could be achieved after just several minutes of administration. It was several years before the guideline committee reconvened, but based on a more extensive literature search, its recommendation for therapy was considerably modified to simply advising a four-hour period of therapy. This is likely to result in far fewer newborns undergoing invasive testing and being unnecessarily placed in an intensive care unit.

Outcome Reporting Bias

We now turn to a type of publication bias in which a study is published but the original study hypothesis is misrepresented in the published report. The aspect of the study that is most susceptible to being changed is in reporting the study outcomes. This has been found to occur when reporting the results of a clinical trial where the prespecified primary (the most important) study outcome is ignored and another outcome is reported as if it had been the preplanned primary outcome. Surprisingly, this phenomenon (technically called "outcome reporting bias") was only first formally studied in 2004 by An-Wen Chan who compared the published reports of randomized controlled trials and what was stated to be the trial's primary and secondary clinical outcomes with the previously declared outcomes in the trial protocol.[11]

When a trial protocol is prepared, the investigators list one or two of the most important clinical outcomes that they hypothesize will be influenced by the therapy under study, based on all the experimental work that has preceded their trial. They also list a longer series of secondary outcomes that are of interest but not considered to be the most important outcomes. These are more in the "if we get lucky" category because compared to the primary outcomes, they are not as well founded in the earlier science. If a therapy is found to influence only a secondary outcome, it is not usually considered to be a definitive demonstration of the therapy's effectiveness.

Astonishingly, Chan found that almost two-thirds of the published reports were discrepant with the stated goals of the trial as written in the protocol: in 34 percent the primary outcome in the protocol was published as a secondary outcome; for 26 percent the protocol's primary outcome was not even reported in the publication; 19 percent of studies changed a secondary outcome in the protocol to make it primary in the report; and 17 percent published as a primary outcome something not even mentioned in the protocol.

Among the examples documented by Chan were trials where the proportion of patients with severe cerebral bleeding was changed from a primary to a secondary outcome, the primary outcome of event-free survival was omitted from the published report, an overall symptom score was changed from a secondary outcome in the protocol to primary in the publication, and the proportion of patients with a graft occlusion was not mentioned in the protocol but listed as the primary outcome in the report. Overall, 50 percent of the efficacy outcomes listed in the protocol and 65 percent of the harm outcomes were incompletely reported in the publication. Why is this important? Having read this far into the book, readers will not be surprised to learn that the statistically significant outcomes were being reported in a disproportionate manner; in fact, statistically significant outcomes pertaining to the effectiveness of the treatment were almost two and a half times more likely to be reported than nonsignificant ones. For the outcomes concerning possible harm from the therapy, the bias was even higher: statistically significant outcomes were almost five times more likely to be reported than nonsignificant ones.

It is axiomatic in science that a specific intervention is *predicted* to cause a precise outcome or event. This is described in the hypothesis being tested and there is no room for variability. The hypothesis must be tested, and then based on the data it will be rejected or not rejected (it cannot be formally proven, see chapter 6, but we can informally say it has been "accepted"). If the hypothesis is accepted, it becomes a building block toward a more general theory of the phenomenon under study. If the hypothesis is rejected, new hypotheses are proposed for future testing. If the primary hypothesized outcome was not statistically significant but another outcome was, then the hypothesis has been rejected and a new hypothesis concerning the successful outcome can be proposed. The difference is not subtle: a new hypothesis cannot be accepted in a study of a prior hypothesis, the new hypothesis can only be *generated*. It must be tested in a new study. What Chan uncovered was the deliberate perversion of the scientific process by relabeling what may well have been a spurious but statistically significant finding as if it were testing a primary hypothesis.[12]

Stephen Jay Gould, the Harvard evolutionary biologist, pointed to the invidious effect of publication bias on the scientific process: "In publication bias, prejudices arising from hope, cultural expectation, or the definitions of a particular theory dictate that only certain kinds of data will be viewed as worthy of publication, or even of documentation at all. Publication bias bears no relationship whatever with the simply immoral practice of fraud; but paradoxically, publication bias may exert a far more serious effect (largely because the phenomenon must be so much more common than fraud)—for scientists affected by publication bias do not recognize their errors (and their bias may be widely shared among colleagues), while a perpetrator of fraud operates with conscious intent, and the wrath of a colleague will be tremendous upon any discovery."[13] Disappointingly, Chan found that 86 percent of authors denied any existence of unreported outcomes despite clear evidence to the contrary in the protocol.

In the study of antidepressants, described earlier in this chapter, it was also noted that the methods sections in 11 of the 37 published papers differed from the prespecified methods described for the FDA. In every study, a positive result was reported as being the primary outcome. When the prespecified primary outcome was reported as being negative, in two reports it was relegated to having a secondary status or it was completely omitted (in nine reports).[14]

Duplicitous and Duplicate Publication

When scientists submit a paper for publication they must assure the journal's editor that the paper has not been previously published and that it is not being considered for publication by any other journal. The intent is to avoid essentially identical reports from entering the research literature. The reasons for this are twofold. Elsewhere we have discussed the importance of replication as a tool for validating research findings; this implies that the replicate research projects are independent of each other. Ideally they involve different investigators, but certainly they must include unique study subjects. There are differing degrees of duplication, ranging from the egregious examples of the same paper being published in more than one journal—usually reflecting an effort (that almost always fails) to pad an academic curriculum vitae, to the appearance of the same study subjects, sometimes innocently, in multiple study reports. The former is more properly called "duplicitous publication," and we will discuss several examples of duplicity and duplication below.

One common duplicitous strategy is to publish a paper in another language and then to republish in English, or vice versa, sometimes with a rearrangement of the author list. When I confronted the French author of a paper that had been republished in English, I was told it was for two reasons, both specious—to give another author a chance at first authorship and to make the paper more widely available. An author deserves to be listed first on a paper only if he or she earned it, by leading the research; the language is irrelevant. Moreover, there are ways of highlighting the work of two authors that is considered of equal importance (these were not used in this paper). Further, the availability of electronic databases makes almost all the world's research literature available. It is revealing that in this example the earlier French publication was not cited in the later English one, making it questionable whether the English editor was informed of the existence of the earlier publication.[15]

How common is duplicate publication? This has been examined in a website creatively named Déjà Vu that collects examples of publication duplication although the website editors seem more interested in the duplicitous variety. In one analysis of a sample of 62,213 citations in MEDLINE using software for comparing text, 1.35 percent of papers with the same authors were judged to be duplicates and 0.04 percent had different authors, raising the specter of possible plagiarism.[16] Less duplicitous examples of publication duplication are more difficult to identify, but they pose problems for scholars trying to synthesize research literature or conducting meta-analyses.

Pregnant women who are epileptic need to be medicated to control their epilepsy symptoms, but the obvious question arises: does this incur complication to the fetus from the therapy? Since only about 1 percent of pregnant women are epileptic and congenital malformations are rare, the usual research practice is to examine the records of birth defect registries. In 1999 a Dr. F. J. E. Vajda and colleagues founded the Australian Register of Antiepileptic Drugs in Pregnancy to address this question, and since then at least half a dozen papers have been published from the accumulating data in the registry.[17] There is nothing improper about the regular publication of data from registries of this type provided prior publications are cited and the authors are always explicit about their earlier work, as the Australian investigators are. Indeed, it is laudable that they are trying to keep the published information from the registry as current as possible. However, researchers who are synthesizing research data need to be aware that the birth defects cases reported in the first publications continue to be reported in the later ones; the reports are not independent.

Similar issues arise when the large Scandinavian databases, which are excellent resources for examining the association of rare exposures with uncommon diseases, are used. In 2007, the well-respected epidemiologist Dr. Bengt Källén published a study linking three Swedish registries (births, birth defects, and patients) to examine the question of whether antidepressant drugs when used by pregnant women increased their risk of having a congenitally malformed child. In this publication over 860,000 children were studied. A 2010 study of over 1 million children by Dr. Margareta Reis, a colleague of Dr. Källén and using the same databases, included all the children from the earlier paper. Again, the authors were careful to point this out but careless readers may assume these were two very large and independent studies.[18] Certainly, they have been used in this way, knowingly or not, by unscrupulous expert witnesses for plaintiffs in lawsuits on this matter (disclosure, I have been a consultant on the opposite side). Meta-analysts of these types of study must be aware to include in their analyses only the most recent data from a sequence of reports from the same database.

More difficult to delineate are what appear to be independent reports that may include the same patients. This occurs particularly when rare outcomes are being studied. An interesting group of uncommon cases and their exposures may be written up by hospital staff, the same cases may be reported to a case registry where a different group of doctors include them in a publication of a larger series of cases on the same exposure, and they may also form part of a national data set where the cases are again published—all without reference to the earlier publications. This may have happened in 2007 for two seemingly independent and highly publicized reports published together in the *New England Journal of Medicine* which also examined the risk of congenital malformation in mothers using antidepressants. One study included cases from hospitals in the cities of Boston, New York, and San Diego and the other study used cases from state birth defect registries emanating from Massachusetts, California, and New York, with the time period for births covered in one study fully overlapping the births in the other. It seems highly likely that the cases from the hospitals in one study were also listed in the state registries.[19]

Interest in these types of study, if it is to inform patient management and address issues of causality, has to ultimately focus on specific drugs and examine particular malformations. The evidence for an association invariably rests on a very small number of exposed cases, and the actual number can affect how one views causality. In this example, interest has focused on the drug paroxetine (Paxil) and right ventricular outflow tract obstructive (RVOTO) defects that occur in the heart. The statewide registries reported six babies with RVOTO who had been exposed to paroxetine and the hospital-based study one. Whether this last case was included in the six is unknown but seems likely. If the same cases are being reported in different studies, then there is no longer replication of the observation and an important criterion for causality is lost. This point was not mentioned by the journal's editorial writer in an otherwise perceptive commentary and was also missed, one suspects, by the journal editors themselves. It was certainly not picked up by the journalists covering the story.[20]

The duplication problem arising from the same cases being reported many times in multiple data sets will only increase. There is now a strong mandate for investigators to make their data sets broadly available so that they can be reanalyzed and republished, and genetic data sets are already being publicly archived, repeatedly reanalyzed, and published many times, making it difficult to track their publication history. Scientists will have to pay more attention to the problem of the same data reoccurring in multiple papers when they try to weight the overall evidence for a particular risk association.

In this chapter we have seen that publication bias is a quite frequent phenomenon. Not only does it pervert the scientific process, contributing to the adoption of ineffective and possibly harmful therapies, but it can have fateful consequences. Fortunately, in recent years, recognition of the insidious influence of publication bias has resulted in the creation of electronic databases for the registration of clinical trial protocols. These allow the progress and eventual publication of trial results to be tracked and comparisons made with those study outcomes which were initially proposed in the protocol and what is reported at the end of the study.[21] In observational studies that are examining potential harms, there has been less progress and some opposition to the registration of study protocols although the imperative to do so is no less important.[22]

FIFTEEN

Causes

When you hear hoof beats behind you, think horses not zebras.
—*Anonymous*

Pluralitas non est ponenda sine neccesitate.
—*William of Ockham*

In January 2011, Jared Loughner shot and killed 6 people and critically wounded 13 others, including Representative Gabrielle Giffords, and the editorial pages were full of angst and commentary as to what had caused the tragedy. Supporters of the gun lobby were quick to fault the mental health system, schools were criticized for not reporting the killer's early signs of sickness, political rhetoric was blamed and, of course, his parents. God was praised for causing Ms. Giffords's remarkable recovery but not for preventing the shooting in the first place. An obvious cause was rarely mentioned: a mentally ill person with all the symptoms of paranoid schizophrenia lived in an environment where he had access to an automatic pistol that could shoot 33 rounds in 10 seconds. Every country has people with schizophrenia, and in most of them, like the United States, they live in the community. But if these mentally ill people have a beef with a politician it usually results in an egg being thrown or a punch in the face, not the ballistic mayhem that ensued in a Tucson shopping mall. People, even mentally ill ones, don't cause the deaths of so many others, guns do. As medical students are taught when trying to make a diagnosis, first think about the obvious causes of a patient's symptoms. Hearing hoof beats, a horse is more likely than a zebra. This remains sound advice for those trying to understand causation. The first things to examine should be the obvious ones; zebras do beat their hooves, and unusual, even esoteric causes of disease will occur but look first for the common ones.

William of Ockham's dictum, commonly translated as "keep it simple, stupid" or perhaps, as preferred in the Latin classroom, "plurality should not be assumed without necessity" famously warns us not to accept complex explanatory phenomena when simpler explanations exist. It has been used for centuries to understand and explain many phenomena, including the nonexistence of God. The argument is that God is not necessary to explain life as we understand it; he is an unnecessary hypothesis. William, who was a monk, would not have approved of this extension of his ideas, but Pope John XXII presumably understood the implications and summoned William to Avignon to explain himself. Ockham's is a second principle that still usefully guides scientists trying to understand causes. They might not be where the journey ends, but common and simple explanations should be the first ports of call in any voyage of causal discovery.

The British Civil Service didn't think causality was a simple matter. In 1859, the examination for the British India Service asked a question that would surely stump most members of the modern British Foreign Office or their colleagues in the US State Department: "What Experimental Methods are applicable to the determination of the true antecedent in phenomena where there may be a Plurality of Causes?" The odd placement of capital letters give a clue as to the emphasis placed on experimental methods, which one must applaud, and plurality of causes, which gives a hint as to why the British were a successful colonial power: these servants of empire really understood how complex a business it was to maintain control over one-quarter of the globe.[1]

The people who lived in Times Beach, Missouri, faced a very different threat from those in Tucson. A small town on the banks of the Meramec River, 17 miles west of St. Louis, Times Beach in 1982 was in transition from a weekend cottage community to a neighborhood of permanent homes. It also had very dusty roads. Marilyn Leistner, who describes herself as the last mayor of Times Beach, tells the story.[2] The town hired Russell Bliss, a waste oil hauler, to spray the roads in the summer of 1972 and 1973. Ten years later, a reporter informed the city that they may have been sprayed with waste oil contaminated with dioxin, and the Environmental Protection Agency confirmed the story. Not surprisingly, the people in the town were desperate for information, were concerned about their own and their children's health, and were of many opinions as to which remedies they should seek. Only a few weeks later the city suffered severe flooding, and on December 23 the town's people received what they called their Christmas message "If you are in town it is advisable for you to leave and if you are out of town do not go back." The former mayor says the community was transformed overnight into a national symbol of something uninhabitable.

On February 22, 1983, the Environmental Protection Agency issued a press release announcing that dioxin had been found at levels ranging from undetectable to 100 ppb and that the town would be permanently relocated.[3] Given such a drastic and disruptive solution to a perceived risk to health caused by dioxin, what was the evidence for health effects? Dioxin, an herbicide, is a widely studied chemical that was used from 1962 to 1971 by US military forces during the Vietnam War to defoliate forests that could conceal their enemy, the Viet Cong. Because of uncertainty about the long-term health effects to the US soldiers, in 1991 Congress passed the Agent Orange Act requiring a biannual review of the state of knowledge about dioxin and health by the Institute of Medicine (IOM), a widely respected and authoritative body of independent scientists.

The state of knowledge in 1982 is best understood by the reports from the IOM committees in the last decade. There is far from any certainty that dioxin had any negative health effects on the US soldiers and airmen, many of whom were exposed to much higher amounts than the residents of Times Beach. Not only did the IOM committees fail to find evidence that dioxin caused health effects, they were not sure there was even any association. The IOM updated their report in 2006: "A Veterans and Agent Orange Committee found itself deadlocked on several of the health outcomes, and were unable to come to a consensus on their categorization. As a result, the health outcomes were left in the category of inadequate or insufficient evidence of an association."[4] In the 2008 report it was concluded that there was "suggestive but limited evidence that exposure to Agent Orange and other herbicides during the Vietnam War is associated with an increased chance of developing ischemic heart disease and Parkinson's disease."[5] The risks for cancer remained uncertain and ranged from EPA estimates that environmental dioxin caused an additional 400 cancer deaths nationally per year in the United States to another conclusion that dioxin did not incur any additional cancer deaths from any dioxin exposure, including that taken in by diet (by far the most common source of human exposure).[6]

Times Beach is a cautionary tale in many respects: bureaucratic confusion is evident as is overreach from an agency that was poorly prepared to manage the ensuing crisis and failed to understand the far-reaching consequences of its actions. Many of the Times Beach residents will understandably attribute their health problems to the dioxin in their environment, just as many veterans of the Vietnam War blamed dioxin for their subsequent health problems, and both groups can make an argument that they should be compensated for the disruptions to their lives caused by governmental action. But none of this provides reliable scientific evidence for a causal association. The health effects of dioxin remain uncertain, although we do know that if there are any increased risks, they are exceedingly small and must affect only a tiny proportion of exposed individuals. In the ten years between spraying oil and discovering it was contaminated with dioxin, there was no discernible change in the health of the Times Beach residents. Had they been spared a massive and stressful upheaval, it seems almost certain that their health would have continued to be unaffected by their exposure.

The preceding two examples showed confusion over causation—from Tucson, which would have benefited from Ockham's razor to point to the obvious, and Times Beach, where an overzealous agency instituted draconian measures to manage an environmental exposure for which no evidence for causation existed. Let us now turn to another cautionary tale, that of thalidomide and Frances Kelsey.

A Canadian by birth and trained in Chicago, Dr. Frances Kelsey had been at the FDA for only a few months, working as a drug safety officer, when she was asked to consider an application for Kevadon (now better known as thalidomide) from the manufacturer, Richardson-Merrell. The drug was already approved as a tranquilizer and sedative in most European countries and Canada, and the manufacturer was bringing considerable pressure on the FDA for approval in the United States. Dr. Kelsey had read reports of peripheral neuritis following use of the drug, suggesting to her there were toxic effects, and so she delayed approving the drug, demanding more evidence of safety. In so doing, she prevented hundreds and possibly thousands of children being born with substantial deformities to their limbs, making her one of the heroines of public health.

Thalidomide had first been introduced, in 1956, in Germany, and it became one of the most widely used of all drugs, being sold without the need of a prescription and used by pregnant women to treat early morning nausea. This most often occurs in the first trimester, the period when the fetal organs are still forming and so are particularly susceptible to any teratogenic effects of drugs. An Australian doctor, W. G. McBride, was the first to make a connection between the birth defect phocomelia and the mother's use of thalidomide. Phocomelia is characterized by failure of the limb buds to develop, and a child exposed to thalidomide in utero is born with one to four undeveloped limbs. Eventually over 10,000 children were born with this condition and virtually all of them resulted from exposure to the drug. Phocomelia is also a genetic condition and under normal circumstances is seen in fewer than 1 per 5,000 births; however, among mothers who used thalidomide some 30 percent had phocomelia,[7] a relative increased risk of 1,500-fold. This is such a high increased risk that causality could be assumed, even though the studies documenting it were poorly controlled and are deficient in all the criteria normally needed to support a conclusion of causality based on smaller increased risks.

Formal Constructs of Causation

The Postulates of Dr. Koch

Robert Koch, a researcher into the causes of anthrax and tuberculosis in the late nineteenth century, was the first to formally outline a set of criteria that would define a causal agent for a disease. Given the infectious nature of the diseases he was investigating, it is not surprising that his focus was on the microorganisms responsible for disease. His four criteria are:

1. The microorganism must be abundant in those suffering from the disease but absent in healthy people.

2. The microorganism can be isolated from a diseased organism and grown in pure culture.
3. The cultured microorganism should cause disease when introduced into a healthy organism.
4. The microorganism must be re-isolated from the inoculated, diseased experimental host and be identical to the specific causative agent.

Koch himself recognized the postulates were imperfect. The first postulate was disproven when cholera bacteria were found in asymptomatic subjects, and now it is known that most infectious disease, such as influenza, HIV, and poliomyelitis, infect many patients who do not exhibit any symptoms of the disease. The third postulate quite often fails when a healthy organism does not become diseased despite being infected. Nonetheless, if an agent does meet the four postulates, it is considered to prove a causal link between the agent and the disease, but not meeting the criteria does not mean that causation is ruled out. The postulates are sufficient but not necessary to prove infectious disease causation. However, they are not useful for noninfectious (also called chronic) diseases, which led Bradford Hill, about whom we had more to say in chapters 4 and 6, to develop his criteria.

The Criteria of Bradford Hill

If there were an epidemiology bible, Sir Austin Bradford Hill would surely be its Moses and his criteria the "ten commandments," although there are only nine of them and his tablet was a paper delivered to the Royal Society of Medicine in 1965. Hill's paper, "The Environment and Disease: Association or Causation," remains the most widely cited set of criteria for establishing that an observed association between an environmental exposure and a disease is likely causal.[8] His criteria appear to be listed in no particular order, and Hill suggests that number 8 (Experiment) is the strongest of them. Here they are listed in their original order, with some of Hill's original examples:

1. *Strength of Association.* It is clear from what he has written elsewhere in his paper that Hill is referring to the relative risk

as the measure of association, and he provides as examples the work of eighteenth-century surgeon Percivall Pott (1714–1788), who found a multifold increase of scrotal cancer in chimney sweeps compared to children not so occupied (children were required to climb up the chimneys to brush them clean), a risk that Richard Doll later estimated was at least 200 times greater than normal. John Snow (1813–1858), the English physician and epidemiologist, is also referenced as having demonstrated a fourteen-fold greater risk of cholera among the inhabitants of homes supplied by the polluted water of the Southwark and Vauxhall Company compared to those drinking the "sewage free" water of the Lambeth Company. Hill also points to his own previous work with Doll that showed increased relative risks of 8, 20, and 32 for lung cancer among smokers versus nonsmokers, increasing with the number of cigarettes smoked. Nonetheless, Hill warns that smaller relative risks may also be present in a causal relationship. He doesn't say how small, but some examples are discussed elsewhere in this book (for example, smoking and myocardial infarction which has a relative risk of between 2 and 3).

2. *Consistency.* Hill's description of this as an association having "been repeatedly observed by different persons, in different places, circumstances and times" suggests he is referring to what today is more commonly called "replication" (see chapter 13). There is no comment as to how many replications are preferable, but the example Hill gives of 36 replications of the smoking–lung cancer association suggests he means more than two or three.

3. *Specificity.* This criterion refers to the association of the environmental agent being "limited to specific workers and to particular sites and types of disease." However, it is now widely recognized that a lack of specificity does not rule out causality, and Hill himself recognized that smoking resulted in a variety of diseases.

4. *Temporality.* Hill describes this as the horse-and-cart problem: which came first? His example of whether different dietary

components cause disease or whether disease influences diet remains a contentious problem to this day. Temporality is discussed throughout this book using the modern concept of reverse causality, but irrespective of what it is called, temporality is one of the necessary criteria for establishing a causal association. Temporality can be wildly misleading: "Post hoc, ergo propter hoc" is one of the oldest of all maxims warning against assuming that just because one event followed another it was necessarily caused by it. Teasing out the correct temporal sequence can be a very tricky exercise.

5. *Biological gradient.* This is the dose response criterion that requires increased risk with greater exposure to the environmental agent. It is discussed in more detail, including why it may be misleading, in the chapter on studies of harm. Nonetheless, the demonstration of a risk gradient according to dose of exposure is still considered a powerful indication of causality.

6. *Plausibility.* Hill describes this as a "helpful" criterion because he realized that it depended on the state of biological knowledge, which is always incomplete. He knew from his own work that the biological basis for smoking and cancer was inadequate for developing a plausible argument sufficient to support a causal association. A biological basis for why smoking causes lung cancer has been formulated in great detail only in recent years. Hill also realized that epidemiological research is able to show strong associations before any other scientific discipline has had the chance to marshal evidence about the biology supporting the association.

7. *Coherence.* This is the other side of the plausibility coin: the observed association should not conflict with what is known about the biology and natural history of the disease. Again, Hill uses smoking as an example, specifically the increase in smoking with a concomitant rise in lung cancer deaths. In line with the greater frequency of smoking among men, they experienced a higher death rate than women. This criterion

does not have the same self-critical appraisal from Hill that is seen elsewhere in his paper. We now know, and it was surely not unknown in 1965, that so-called ecological correlations between a changing environment over time and increasing (or decreasing) disease incidence can be quite misleading.

8. *Experiment.* This is the criterion described by Hill as possibly revealing the strongest support for causation. In particular, if it can be accomplished, does removal of the environmental agent lead to a decrease in the risk of disease? If these criteria were commandments, number eight would be the Golden Rule (do unto others as you would have done unto you). Modern epidemiologists who are investigating an association will always first try to see if an experimental research design is possible, using a randomized controlled trial. Unlike Goldberger's experiment with the pellagra-inducing diet in prisoners, experiments to see whether an agent actually causes harm are widely considered to be unethical and are rarely done. Thus this golden criterion is actually unavailable to investigators studying harm, and causality often remains an uncertain conclusion.

9. *Analogy.* Hill uses the thalidomide and rubella examples, which were topical when he was writing, to make his point: "We would surely be ready to accept slighter but similar evidence with another drug or another viral disease in pregnancy." But this criterion is now recognized to be flawed. It has resulted in many useful drugs and contraceptives being removed from the pharmacopeia because of premature and incorrect conclusions that they were causing health problems. Classes of drugs and chemicals, such as hormones, solvents, and even asbestos, include specific typologies within the class that have very different risk profiles, including no risk, for disease. Kenneth Rothman, author of some of the most influential textbooks written for epidemiology students, had this to say about analogy: "Whatever insight might be derived from analogy is handicapped by the inventive imagination of scientists who can find analogies everywhere."[9]

It is another aspect of Hill's lack of insight on this aspect of his own paper that he allowed himself to comment: "Thus on relatively slight evidence we might decide to restrict the use of a drug for early-morning sickness in pregnant women. If we are wrong in deducing causation from association no great harm will be done. The good lady and the pharmaceutical industry will doubtless survive." Hill had obviously never suffered from morning sickness, but his misogynistic comment, which was clearly made with the thalidomide disaster in mind, would have ramifications for another anti-emetic, Bendectin, in the next decade. This effective and safe therapy was needlessly forced off the market by remorseless litigation leaving to this day women without adequately studied drugs to treat their morning sickness (chapter 6 offers a detailed account).

How have Bradford Hill's criteria survived half a century of application? Hill did not consider all the criteria to be necessary for a conclusion of causality to be reached. He observed, "What they can do, with greater or less strength, is to help us make up our minds on the fundamental question — is there any other way of explaining the set of facts before us, is there any other answer equally, or more likely, than cause and effect?" Today, this is how the criteria are generally applied: analogy and coherence are widely ignored; plausibility is often derived from animal studies, which are increasingly seen to be unreliable predictors of human experience (chapter 11), specificity is often not seen; and experimental evidence of harm is usually unavailable. Of the original criteria, only four — the strength of association, temporality, dose, and consistency (replicability) — are considered crucial to demonstrating causation. Another criterion, not mentioned and probably unknown to Hill, might be added: that the association has not suffered from the series of problems known as publication bias, discussed in detail in chapter 14.[10]

Causation in Law

Epidemiology studies usually form a crucial part of the evidence used in toxic tort and medical malpractice litigation, but the construct for causation in the law differs radically from the scientific paradigm. This often leads to confusion when the two professions meet up in the courtroom. Anthony

Barton, a British legal scholar, has written thoughtfully about this and much of what follows is summarized from his writing.[11]

Barton says: "The major distinction between legal determinations and scientific assertions lies in the concept of certainty. The legal concept of causation is deterministic: it is an expression of fiction of certainty, an absolute concept. The scientific concept of causation is probabilistic: it is an expression of the uncertainty of truth, an asymptotic concept."[12] Evidence and proof of causation differ between the two professions: in science, the probabilities of interest are those arising from a study testing a hypothesis; in law, the probability refers to whether the hypothesis itself is true. Scientists are willing to accept uncertainty and suspend judgment if the available data does not allow firm conclusions to be drawn. The law, however, must arrive at a conclusion within the time frame of a trial and the evidence tendered. Uncertainty is not a final option. Justice Blackman, in his *Daubert* decision in the Bendectin litigation, opined: "Scientific conclusions are subject to perpetual revision. Law, on the other hand, must resolve disputes finally and quickly . . . rules of evidence [were] designed not for the exhaustive search for cosmic understanding but for the particularized resolution of legal disputes."[13]

Courts expect the testifying expert witness to use the criteria for causation relevant to their scientific discipline, but this will not be accepted as the standard of proof in the trial. Two legal principles take precedence: the "but for" test and the doctrine of "material contribution." "But for" requires proof that the event under dispute, say a cancer diagnosis, would not have occurred but for the exposure, say to solvents in the workplace. This is a difficult burden for plaintiffs as cancer usually occurs in the absence of solvent exposure and there will be other risk factors for it, not least genetic susceptibility. "Material contribution" refers to the multiple causes of a condition. In law, the plaintiff does not have to show that all possible causes of a condition were the responsibility of a defendant; it is sufficient for the factor at issue in the case to be shown to be a "material" contributing cause to the disease. These principles have been the subject of considerable scholarship in legal circles, but for our purposes it is sufficient to appreciate that entirely different concepts of causation are being applied. Further, these are constructs of general causation, they apply as a general rule: is a chemical capable of causing this disease? General causation has been the focus of this book. However, in law individual causation must also be proved. It may have been accepted as a generality that a drug can cause congenital malformations, but did this plaintiff consume the drug, was it in a sufficiently large dose or at the appropriate time in gestation to cause a malformation, and are there other exposures that may have been more likely to cause the malformation such as a family history?

Science and the courts also differ on their interpretation of risk for general causation. It is widely recognized that a relative risk of 2 or more, at least a doubling of risk, is taken by the courts to be equivalent to the legal standard of "more likely than not," also known as the "51 percent probability rule." This differs from the scientific approach where neither a relative risk of 2.0, nor indeed any size of relative risk, is imbued with such a powerful inference. It is possible that relative risks below 2 meet the criteria for causality, and it is commonplace for relative risks well above 2 to fail to do so. Science also looks for standards of proof well beyond 51 percent, a criterion that is obviously barely distinguishable from chance. If the same legal standard were adopted by scientists, it would destroy the scientific enterprise as numerous false leads were followed. As described elsewhere (chapter 8), typical standards in scientific hypothesis testing are between 90 and 99 percent, with 95 percent being the most widely used level of probability for rejecting the null hypothesis of there being no association. However, these probabilities serve different purposes. The scientific probability is used for testing a hypothesis under the conditions of how a particular study was designed; while the legal test is based on all the available evidence, including the scientific, that causation has been proved.

A Simple Paradigm for Deciding Whether Risk Factors Are Likely Causal

If causation is approached from a practical perspective that takes its cue from those risk factor associations accepted, over the course of decades and much debate, as being causal, there are two overriding considerations that appear to trump all others. First, the size of the association whereby exposure to the agent of interest increases the risk of disease relative to the unexposed; and second, the strength (validity) of the evidence base on which the risk assessment is based and how often the estimate of increased risk has been replicated. Where the evidence for an association is derived from a methodologically weak study, a much larger association is required for evidence of causality. Smaller associations may be causal if they are replicated in methodologically strong studies. An additional critical assumption for the strength of evidence is that the temporal sequence is appropriate for causal interpretation: the exposure must be known to have occurred before the onset of disease. Very large associations that are the product of reverse causation are rare but not unknown, many being the consequences of disease and not causes of them. For example, type 2 diabetes is strongly associated with hypertension; however, whether hypertension is involved in the etiology of diabetes, or is a consequence of it, or whether both share the same underlying pathology that play a role in the onset of both conditions, remains uncertain. These types of strongly associated but not necessarily causal risk factors may be useful in prediction models, described below, but they do not necessarily indicate causality.

Figure 15.1 shows some examples of well-accepted causal associations (the numbers in parentheses, below, refer to the numbers in the figure, which are positioned at approximately the cross-referent point of increased risk and an estimate of the literature's validity and replication of results). Studies linking thalidomide (5), Accutane (11), and sodium valproate (2) to specific congenital malformations are all based on quite small and poorly controlled although replicated case series. All demonstrate very large increases in risk, in the order of 10 to 15 times for sodium valproate and spina bifida and higher for the other two. These results have been observed in many studies, and it is now broadly agreed that the associations are causal. The association of smoking and lung cancer (1) is of similar order of magnitude but has been observed in studies of higher quality and replicated many times. In contrast, the risk of heart disease from smoking (8) is increased only two- to threefold, but the higher-quality research on which it is based and the multiple replications also indicate causality. The association of the

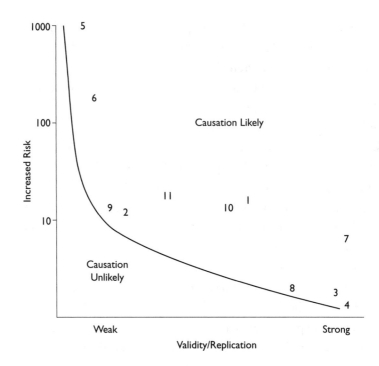

Figure 15.1. A proposal for assessing the likelihood of observing a causal association based on the size of increased risk and the degree of validity and replication. See text for explanation of numbers.

nonsteroidal anti-inflammatory drug Vioxx and myocardial infarction (3) is increased by only about 130 percent (RR = 2.3), but it is based on evidence from a meta-analysis of many randomized trials that obtained similar results. The small increased risk is compensated by the high-validity trials on which it is based and so it is also likely to be causal.

In 1979, the *New England Journal of Medicine* published a study reporting that women who used estrogen were 12 times more likely to develop endometrial cancer than nonusers. The findings were disputed by other investigators on the grounds that estrogens were a cause of vaginal bleeding in some women which would bring them to the attention of doctors and more testing, leading to an earlier diagnosis (what was described as disease

ascertainment bias in chapter 6). This bias was assessed in a study of autopsy data that was itself flawed (*lifetime* risk was calculated for the autopsy
data and compared with *annual* risk for the tumor registry data), suggesting
that there were as many as four times the number of undiagnosed versus
diagnosed cancer cases. When the corrected risks were standardized to the
same time unit, only 20 percent of endometrial cases were undiagnosed.
Ascertainment bias only slightly reduced the increased relative risk for endometrial cancer after estrogen use from 12 to 11.6 (10), still strong enough
to indicate a likely causal relationship.[14]

The corollary of this paradigm is that studies of poor design, such as case
series with inappropriate control groups, and other types of observational research that have not managed to avoid the many biases that jeopardize them
have not historically been able to document causality for relative risks of 1.5
to 5 and rarely in the 6 to 8 range. A very different picture emerges from
genetic studies. These are often free of bias because of genetic recombina-
tion at fertilization (what has been called Mendelian randomization and
is discussed in chapter 6) that should equalize environmental and lifestyle
confounding factors across people with different genetic variations. Adult
macular degeneration (AMD), a form of blindness often affecting people in
their middle age, was associated with a more than 7 times increased risk in
people who had two copies of a risk allele in the compliment factor H gene
(7). The strong methodology of the original genetic study, and subsequent
replication in numerous other well-designed studies, strongly supported a
causal explanation for this association. In other cases, quite small measures
of genetic risk (reduced or increased), even less than 50 percent (RR < 1.50)
may be considered causal if the risks have been replicated in several high-
quality independent studies. Five studies examined whether a polymorphism (238G→A) in a tumor necrosis factor gene (*TNFA*) and meta-analysis
of them demonstrated an increased risk of alcoholic liver cirrhosis (OR =
1.47 95%CI 1.05, 2.07), which is supportive of a causal association (4).[15]

Finally, it is of interest to note two historical associations and where they
fit on this schema. We saw above that cholera was 14 times more likely in
the homes supplied by the suspected water in Hill's analysis of the London

cholera epidemic (9) and Doll's calculation that the eighteenth-century children cleaning chimneys were some 200 times more likely to develop scrotal cancer (6). The methodology from these early epidemiology observations would not meet modern standards; nonetheless, the size of the increased risk provides compelling evidence for a causal association.

The associations above the curved line in figure 15.1 are a few examples of well-documented causal relationships, but what is below the line where causation is labeled as being unlikely? There are thousands of associations presently being studied between almost every environmental and lifestyle factor known to humankind and all the diseases to which we are subject. These associations are either well studied and have not to date produced valid evidence of causality, or they are poorly studied and the evidence is conflicting, or the association is just beginning to be investigated and not enough well-designed and replicated research has been completed. As new chemicals and compounds are developed, novel drugs are designed, innovative technologies enter our lives, and different behavior patterns are adopted, questions about their potential health effects always arise. Special plastics and gene therapies, cell phones and running marathons into middle and older age have all emerged in the last 20 years. A complete profile of what health risks they may cause, if any, remains uncertain. Experience tells us that the vast majority of associations presently being studied will prove to be harmless, although not a small number will be subject to false alarms and even crusades against them, as described elsewhere in this book. Nonetheless, because of the large number of people exposed to possible harm and the substantial negative effects on health that some exposures may incur, it is necessary to examine the possible role of all of them in causing disease. This, as we have discussed, is the science of epidemiology and as problematic as it can sometimes be to document causality, it remains by far our most successful methodology for uncovering causal relationships.

A sampling of associations currently being examined by epidemiologists points to their great diversity. All the examples listed below were presented at the Third North American Congress of Epidemiology, held in Montreal in June 2011. Some of the associations studied suggest risks but others protective effects or no risk. For the most part, this is work in progress, and the final conclusions about whether these are causal associations, at the time of this writing, remains undetermined.

DDT and liver cancer

Coffee or tea (or red meat) and colorectal cancer

Bisphenol-A (BPA) and low birth weight and children's neuro-development

Perfluorinated compounds (PFCs) and subfertility

Organophosphate insecticides and wheezing

Risk factors for total knee replacement failure

Effect of alcohol consumption on HIV acquisition

Hurricane Katrina experience and risk of gestational diabetes

Residential proximity to power transmission lines and stillbirth

Higher environmental temperature during pregnancy and low birth weight

Fish consumption and depression

In utero exposure to diagnostic radiation and childhood cancer

Isoflavones (phytoestrogens) and breast cancer

Vitamin and calcium supplements and breast cancer survival or recurrence

Mobile phone use and acoustic neuroma

More Complex Models of Causality

Very large increases in risk provide a reliable clue as to whether a single association is likely to prove causal, even among epidemiological studies plagued by bias. Smaller increases in risk may be documented as causal when derived from methodologically strong studies, for example, randomized trials and well-controlled genetic studies. But these associations are rarely themselves able to fully explain disease causation. Disease is not usually caused by a single agent, and to understand the complex interplay of the many interacting factors usually needed to produce disease, more complex causal models are required. Columbia University professor of epidemiology

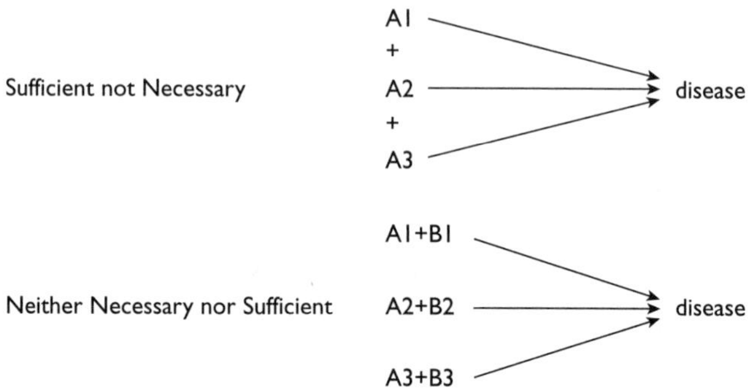

Figure 15.2. A model of causation: concepts of necessity and sufficiency.

Mervyn Susser has written thoughtfully on concepts of causality that incorporate the ideas of necessity and sufficiency.[16] He describes four typologies, for any single risk factor, and these are schematized in figure 15.2.

1. *The risk factor is necessary and sufficient.* This is a situation that only rarely applies: head trauma is induced by a single blow to the cranium and paralysis after acute spinal injury follows from a vigorous tackle on the football field. An extra chromosome 21, which involves a massive amount of additional DNA, always results in symptoms characteristic of Down syndrome (although the severity can vary). However, variations at the level of a single gene, such as the breast cancer genes *BRCA1* and *BRCA2*, frequently, but by no means always, cause disease. In one study, 28 percent of women with the *BRCA1* variant had developed breast cancer by age 50 and 84 percent by age 70.[17] Most major genetic variants are rarely sufficient for disease to inevitably follow. Even agents causing quite contagious diseases are rarely sufficient to always cause symptoms of

disease. Because of the use of AIDS drugs it is difficult to derive current estimates of how many HIV positive persons actually develop AIDS, but this is also influenced by other factors such as age, other infections, and nutritional status. Children born HIV positive because of infection from the mother during birth provide one estimate of how frequently AIDS develops. In one large study, by age five, 40 to 50 percent of them had not developed symptoms of AIDS.[18]

2. *The risk factor is necessary but not sufficient.* Many infectious disease agents produce symptomatic cases in only a small proportion of those infected: for example, of every 200 persons carrying the polio virus only one will show the characteristic signs of paralysis. This is an important reason why widespread population vaccination is necessary to eradicate this disease. During an influenza epidemic almost every member of the population will show signs of being infected if their blood is examined, but many remain symptom free. Flu may be symptomatic only in patients who are deficient in a nutrient or in people carrying a gene that increases risk. Many genetic variants increase susceptibility but quite often do not always produce disease (as described above, they have low "penetrance"). Schizophrenia almost certainly has a genetic cause, but the symptoms may only be expressed in an environment where another risk factor—possibly another genetic variant, an environmental agent, or a sociocultural condition—is also present.

3. *Each risk factor is sufficient but not necessary.* If several risk factors are all capable of causing disease, then no single one is necessary. Depression may result from many genetic, environmental, and lifestyle causes. Bereavement, post-pregnancy, or other dispiriting life situations may result in clinical depression independent of any known genetic variants. However, susceptibility for many complex diseases, such as cancer, heart disease, autism, or asthma, is almost certainly increased by a large

number of genetic variants, perhaps hundreds of them for each
specific disease. Each gene has a small individual effect on risk
and may work independently of the others.

4. *Each risk factor is neither necessary nor sufficient.* This is the
paradigm that Susser thought would probably apply to most
diseases. In essence, there are multiple independent causal
pathways to the same disease. For example, a genetic variant
may exert its effect only in the presence of other risk factors—
perhaps environmental agents or other genes—to form one
pathway. Another gene variant, in the presence of other environmental factors, may support another pathway to the same
disease. This seems as if it may be the situation for complex
diseases, such as asthma, many cancers, and autism spectrum
disorders. However, these are also conditions where the disease
is actually a mix of multiple and possibly quite different pathological conditions, and this may explain the many possible
causal pathways. As a disease "phenotype" is deconstructed into
discrete entities, it is possible that each one will be explained
by a somewhat simpler causal pathway.

Multifactorial models of disease causation are widely held to be the appropriate paradigm for studying the causes of complex, chronic disease. All
the potential biases that jeopardize research using the simpler constructs of
single risk factor etiology, discussed throughout this book, apply with even
greater force when multiple factors are considered. For example, confounding factors that are linked to both the disease and the exposure of interest now must be associated with several environmental agents. Control of
multifactorial confounding poses great challenges in observational research
studies.

Finally, we should note that causation is not the same as prediction, although these two ideas are frequently confused. It is possible to develop a set
of risk factors that will predict a person who is at high risk of disease without
resorting to using any truly causal factors. Consider a person with yellow
fingers, brown teeth, wrinkles, and a bad cough. We would predict, with a

high degree of certainty, they are a likely candidate for being at increased risk of lung cancer. We discussed earlier how yellow fingers are strongly associated with cigarette smoking and the same applies for brown teeth. Wrinkles and coughing are also associated with smoking, but they are a result of smoking, not a cause. Of course, the same "prediction model" would also predict that someone is a smoker. Prediction models can be very useful for characterizing people who may be at particularly high risk for disease, but they should not be confused with causal models. Eliminating the risk factors in a prediction model may have no impact on the frequency of the disease, but eliminating risk factors operating in a true causal model most assuredly will.

SIXTEEN

Ultimate Causation

Allergy warning. Contains mustard.
—*On a jar of Batts English mustard*

Goldberger, Snow, Doll, and many other public health heroes are celebrated for demonstrating causal relationships between dietary deficiencies, polluted drinking water, cigarette smoking, and a host of other factors shown to cause serious disease. Their discoveries were done at a time when it was not known what was ultimately causing the diseases they studied; there were no blindingly obvious labels about disease-causing products, such as a warning on a mustard jar that it contained mustard. Nonetheless, once shown, or in some cases strongly suspected, that an exposure was causal, it was possible to implement relatively straightforward public health actions: adding nutrients to the diet, removing the (perhaps apocryphal) water pump handle, and implementing smoking cessation programs, all of which were sufficient to substantially lower the incidence of disease.[1]

We have discussed in the preceding chapter the concepts of causation proposed by Koch and Bradford Hill and the necessity and sufficiency of risk factors described by Susser. We also noted that predictive models of disease risk are not the same as causal models because many predictive factors may be the result of unrecognized or undiagnosed disease, such as childhood wheeze being predictive of asthma. Causal risk factors must necessarily be antecedent to the onset of the disease they cause. We can invoke three further distinctions in the risk factors that are antecedent to disease: distal, proximal, and ultimate factors.

Distal risk factors are those that are in place long before the disease process is known to begin (although this may reflect our incomplete knowledge of the full natural history of a disease). These include genetic variation that may be present from conception or subsequently as a result of epigenetic change. Other distal causal risk factors may have occurred during the in utero period, perhaps because of maternal starvation or nutritional deficiencies. Gender is a distal risk factor as it incorporates many other important factors (for example, hormonal exposures). Height is another; taller women have recently been shown to be at increased risk for many cancers.[2] Using Susser's paradigm, the distal factors are likely to be neither necessary nor sufficient for disease causation.

Proximal risk factors are those to which exposure occurs closer in time to disease onset. These include chemicals, drugs, and radiation and other types of environmental exposure discussed throughout this book. Viruses, bacteria, and other agents associated with infectious disease are also proximal risk factors. While many proximal risk factors are closely antecedent to the onset of disease, such as the maternal use of drugs causing congenital malformations, others have a delayed effect. Diethylstilbestrol (DES) prescribed to mothers during their pregnancy, in the mistaken belief it would reduce their risk of miscarriage, 20 or more years later caused vaginal adenocarcinoma that was diagnosed in many of their daughters (although how long before diagnosis the disease process started is unclear, perhaps at the time of exposure). Proximal causal factors are most likely either necessary but not sufficient, or sufficient but not necessary, for causing disease.

Finally, there are the ultimate causal risk factors. These are those factors that provide the tipping point for the initiation of the final disease process. Again using Susser's nomenclature, ultimate causal risk factors are likely to be necessary and sufficient to cause disease. In none of the early public health triumphs, as dramatically successful as they were in preventing disease, was the ultimate cause of the disease understood. This matters because successful therapy often depends on a detailed understanding of causal pathways, including the ultimate cause. Screening and diagnosis are also much more effective the further forward along the causal chain are the biological factors being screened. Cholesterol (a distal risk factor) is an inefficient screening tool, but prenatal screening for the additional chromosome number 21 that is synonymous with Down syndrome (an ultimate causal factor) is highly effective. In contrast, preventing disease, as we have seen, can be effective even if based on the distal risk factors that increase risk for disease without necessarily causing it. This is why the pump handle has become the iconic symbol of epidemiology.

The actual nutrient whose deficiency caused pellagra, niacin, and the precise mechanism by which niacin exerts its affect was not understood until many years after Goldberger's death, when in 1935 Conrad Elvehjem (1901–1962), a Norwegian American from Wisconsin, identified nicotinamide as a hydrogen acceptor and donor for many enzymes involved in metabolism. Similarly, Robert Koch (1843–1910) was long thought to have discovered the cholera vibrio in 1884, after putting into practice his postulates described in the previous chapter. However, thirty years earlier Filippo Pacini (1812–1883), professor of anatomy in Florence, published a paper describing the comma-shaped bacillus found in the intestinal mucosa of cholera victims. For our purposes, it is noted that this publication was only four years before John Snow's death and long after his work on the London cholera epidemic. Snow did not know the ultimate cause of cholera. Even identifying the cholera vibrio doesn't fully explain how it causes the disease. Work has continued to explore the effect of the organism on the permeability of the intestinal capillaries and the leakage of fluid that follows, and quite recently the genome of the vibrio was sequenced to identify the genes that bring about this effect. This mechanistic work on cholera continues, but my point has been made. Ultimate causation is difficult to pinpoint and often not necessary for prevention or, as exemplified by cholera, successful treatment.

What is meant by ultimate cause? Aristotle writes about "final cause" or *telos* being the most important of the four causal factors he espoused (the others being material cause, formal cause, and efficient cause); in his example, the final cause of a saw being able to cut wood rests in the iron teeth.[3] This is analogous to how I use the term "ultimate cause." This is not to say that the ultimate cause is necessarily more important than all the antecedent events that set up the ultimate cause and propelled the organism into starting a disease process. Aristotle also recognized that not all phenomena have a known cause, but he did propose the concept that seems most useful for our purposes. The concept of ultimate cause refers to the final, in a temporal sense, causal event that tips the healthy cell (and it usually is a cell or cells) into a state where it becomes a tumor, or causes embryological development to go awry resulting in a birth defect, or induces the immune system to fail to cope with an onslaught of foreign bodies.

The ultimate causative agents for lung cancer are among the 4,000 chemicals found in cigarette smoke, some 60 of which are known carcinogens. The polycyclic aromatic hydrocarbons (PAHs) are among the most potent carcinogens, principal of which is benzo[a]pyrene and the tobacco-specific nitrosamine 4-(methylnitro-samino)-1-(3-pyridyl)-1-butanone. These compounds occur in small quantities, typically about 5–200 ng per cigarette. Somewhat weaker but more prevalent carcinogens are the aldehydes and other volatile organic compounds, such as benzene and butadiene, that are found in quantities of 10–1000 ng per cigarette. Nicotine is not itself carcinogenic but must be considered part of the causal chain because its addictive properties are undoubtedly responsible for more people smoking for longer periods of time than they might wish. Cytochrome P450 enzymes add an oxygen atom to the carcinogens to increase water solubility, DNA adducts are created, and mutations follow resulting in uncontrolled cell growth. The carcinogenic process is well understood and has been described in great detail—and with each step being under genetic control.[4] Again and with some relief, we part company from it here because the point is made. Doll, Hill, Wynder, and Graham, in the 1950s, drew their conclusions that cigarette smoking caused lung cancer without any of the knowledge subsequently developed to explain the mechanisms of action of cigarette smoke. The causal chain for every carcinogenic process is long and detailed and even now for many carcinogens ultimate causation remains uncertain.

A new concept of carcinogenesis is focusing on the role of the many microbes that have evolved symbiotically with humans and which inhabit every part of our body. There are many more genes in these microbes than there are in human cells (perhaps as much as 90 percent of all the functional genes in our body belong to microbes, not us!), and they provide considerable opportunity for mutation and play a role in disease causation. Scientists are now exploring how our microbial genes interact through chemical signals with the human genome. It has been known for several years that people in different parts of the world are hosts to a variety of "microbiomes," which may explain the differences in disease rates in different populations. For example, the Japanese have microbes that specialize in seaweed digestion, but how, or if, these relate to the higher rates of stomach and other intestinal cancers in Japan remains unknown. Clearly the ultimate causes of diseases such as cancer can be extremely complex and have a latency period that may cross generations and will take years to unravel.[5]

Our lack of complete knowledge of the fundamental causal pathways for disease—how thalidomide causes limb reduction defects or why smoking causes lung cancer—is often referred to as a "black box." We have noted the many public health benefits that can accrue from documenting causal associations even absent a detailed explanation of how the exposure actually produces disease; indeed, the great majority of documented causal associations, if not all, are first demonstrated without any firm knowledge of the mechanism for causing disease. Only after the disease association has been demonstrated to be causal is there a sustained effort to understand the ultimate causal process. Moreover, ultimate causation is often a moving target. As a causal pathway is increasingly understood at one level, new questions arise at another. With more complete understanding, the black box doesn't disappear but rather it takes on a new form. The "box," with its connotations of being a tidy package, wrapped and ready to be opened, is an inadequate analogy. Perhaps Russian *matryoshkas* or nesting dolls would be more appropriate, as opening one leads to finding another and opening that one to yet more again. But how many dolls are there? In other words, how long is a causal chain?

To understand this, we can borrow the "Linda problem" from the social psychologists who study the rationality of human decision making. Linda is an imaginary bright young girl with a strong social conscience who hated discrimination. Participants in the experiment are asked what is most probable when Linda grows up. Was she most likely to be: (a) a bank teller or (b) a bank teller and active in the feminist movement? If you answered "b" you are one of the approximately 4 in 5 people who answer this problem incorrectly. The operative word is "probable." Whatever the probability of Linda becoming a bank teller (let's say it is 10 percent), the additional prob-

ability of her being active in the feminist movement (let's say it is 80 percent) reduces the overall probability of that outcome. Probabilities are always multiplied, and in this case outcome "b" has a $0.1 \times 0.8 = 0.08$ or an
8 percent chance of occurring. The social psychologists use this and many
experiments like it to point to the inherent lack of rationality in our decision
making. For us, the example makes a different point.

If a causal chain has many elements and each one has some probability
of less than one of occurring, with each link in the chain, the probability of
the final event is much reduced. For example a causal association having
a chain with five events of 20 percent probability of each occurring ($0.2 \times
0.2 \times 0.2 \times 0.2 \times 0.2$) has only a 3 in 10,000 chance of being completed.
This suggests that most causal chains are likely to be short with only a small
number of intervening links. If a chemical exposure results in the disruption of a molecular pathway in a cell, and the damaged cell interferes with
organ development in a developing fetus, there are likely only a few causal
steps involved. By the same token, if each event has a very high probability
of inducing change at the next step, the probability of the final event is high
(indeed, $1.0 \times 1.0 \times 1.0 \times 1.0 = $ certainty, for an infinite number of events).
In this case, it also seems most likely that the causal chains will be shorter
rather than longer. This is not because they are based on probability but
because a long chain of damaged cells or molecular pathways would likely
have other detrimental effects on the body with concomitant negative selection bias resulting in early lethality. However, this type of damaging causal
chain, if it occurs after the reproductive years of an individual, would not
influence selection and is not removed from the population.

As discussed in the previous chapter, exposure to causal agents does not
always, or even most of the time, result in disease. These exposures are
neither necessary nor sufficient. It is widely known that individual genetic
variation increases (or decreases) susceptibility to disease, and examples
of genes interacting with factors in the environment to enhance disease
risk are being uncovered with increasing frequency. Many more so-called
gene-environment and gene-gene interactions will be discovered, as this
is the subject of much current research. The ultimate cause of all physical and mental disease lies at the biochemical level, and discovering these

fundamental biological processes has important implications for how we screen for disease as well as how we treat it. The closer we are to knowing the ultimate cause of disease, the more specific screening tests can be developed that will have fewer false positive or false negative results.

Ultimate causal agents also permit the use of more specific therapies, what is sometimes called personalized medicine. This becomes possible when an individual's genetic sensitivity to a medicine allows the use of more targeted therapy and the avoidance of medications that result in complications and side effects.

Herceptin is one of a group of cancer drugs called "monoclonal antibodies," and one of the first drugs that can target and lock on to specific types of cancer cells. Normal cells have growth factor receptors to which growth factor proteins attach and help the cell grow. However, some patients have extra copies of a particular cancer-causing gene (called an oncogene) known as *HER2*, which results in the surface of some cancer cells having too much of one protein: human epidermal growth factor receptor 2 (HER2) that is regulated by the *HER2* gene. An excess of the HER2 receptors facilitates cancer growth. Blocking the HER2 receptors with the antibody herceptin reduces the amount of growth factor entering the cancer cell and slows down tumor growth.

Herceptin also accentuates the cancer cell, allowing the body's natural immune system to target and destroy it. Herceptin only blocks receptors in HER2-positive cancers which, to date, have been found in the breast and stomach. Because Herceptin works in a novel way it can be used in conjunction with chemotherapy. It was only by obtaining a deep understanding of the causal pathways for disease that these specific therapies could be developed. As of June 2011, the FDA had approved 22 monoclonal antibodies for specific types of atopic-asthma, cardiovascular disease, autoimmune disease, leukemia, colorectal cancer, psoriasis, multiple sclerosis, macular degeneration, non-Hodgkin's lymphoma, and breast cancer.

While the ultimate causes of most diseases remain to be discovered, have all the distal and proximal causes of disease been identified? Is there anything left to discover? During the twentieth century, many large associations (for example, $RR > 5.0$) between environmental or lifestyle factors and disease have been revealed and have resulted in substantial improvements to health. Smoking cessation alone has added several years to longevity for millions of individuals, and blood pressure and cholesterol reduction have significantly lowered death from cardiovascular disease. Without taking anything away from the enormous success of the work so far, these have been the low-hanging fruit that proved amenable to discovery by the methods of observational epidemiology. Future success, in which much less prevalent exposures must be examined for their role in causing disease, will be considerably more difficult to achieve.

There are many more proximal causes of disease to be discovered, and this is a necessary step before ultimate causation can be identified. The path will be littered with numerous false associations, even when great care is taken in conducting these studies. We have seen that many biases can mislead the search for disease causation and many of the false leads suggest an association of an exposure with a disease. Among all the sciences, the "false positives" in epidemiology may have the greatest opportunity for social disruption and they can actually cause harm. The removal of useful drugs and contraceptives from the pharmacopeia and the elimination of beneficial chemicals from industrial processes all because of unwarranted scares has been documented throughout this text. On the other hand, "false negative" results are also extremely damaging. Tens of thousands of unnecessary deaths have resulted from the inappropriate use of hormone replacement therapy and drugs like Vioxx.

Weaker causal associations of exposures with common disease are more difficult to identify, but when they are properly understood the benefit to public health can be very great. They may offer new insight into the mechanisms of disease causation and so into new ways of treating disease. Other benefits accrue from understanding what may be the (modest) risk of widely used exposures. If regular cell (mobile) telephone use resulted in a tenfold (900 percent) increase in risk of brain tumors, the size of the increase makes it likely that it would already have been discovered. But if the increased risk were 20 percent, it would be much harder to detect with confidence, although given the ubiquitous nature of cell phone usage, it would be a very important risk to detect.[6]

The difficulty in reliably documenting causal associations that are modest in strength has resulted in considerable uncertainties and false declarations that have substantially harmed the public's health. It took too long to appreciate the benefits of antenatal steroids for newborn lung maturation for women in preterm labor and too long to recognize the cardiovascular complications of using Vioxx or the increased cancer risk from hormone replacement therapy. Increasingly, epidemiologists are concerned about the safety of rare exposures and whether they cause relatively uncommon outcomes. These are extraordinarily difficult problems to solve, requiring large studies and creative research designs.

Epidemiologists must use the search for association between rare exposure and disease as an opportunity for improving their science. The search for causes will require more attention to experimental detail than heretofore, much more control over the publication process, and a greater willingness to accept uncertainty before declaring that causality has been established. The failure of randomized trials to support long-held beliefs originating from observational studies—the harm caused by combined postmenopausal estrogen use, the failure of low-fat diets to protect against heart disease and cancer, the failure of calcium supplementation to protect against fractures in elderly women, and the increased risk of cancer in some people after beta carotene supplementation, which was thought to protect against cancer—must give pause for reflection as to what went wrong in a large number of epidemiology studies. Observational epidemiology is the only scientific methodology we have for exploring the possible causality of everyday life exposures with health outcomes. Used properly it places very powerful tools at our disposal, but misused it can lead to substantial misinformation and harm.

A Cone of Causation

Previous writers have discussed a "web" of causation to describe the multifactorial causes of disease, and many imaginative and creative efforts have been made to diagram the causal web: Google "images" is a rich source of earlier examples. What is striking about many of them is the absence of any parameter for time, which surely misses a crucial aspect in thinking about how the many factors involved in causation must interact. If we think of what results in, at some particular point in time, a melanoma cell mutating, then some (presently unknown) ultimate causal event must immediately precede it. The distal and proximal events, such as, respectively, fair skin and severe sunburn, are earlier in the causal chain. However, the web is a useful construct,[7] and combining it with a temporal component produces a cone of causation, shown schematically in figure 16.1. It is cone shaped because there are many more distal factors involved with disease susceptibility, exerting their influence earlier in time, than there are factors that function as proximal or ultimate causes.

Figure 16.1 also shows the "induction periods," which are the time that it takes for each causal risk factor to induce the next step in the disease

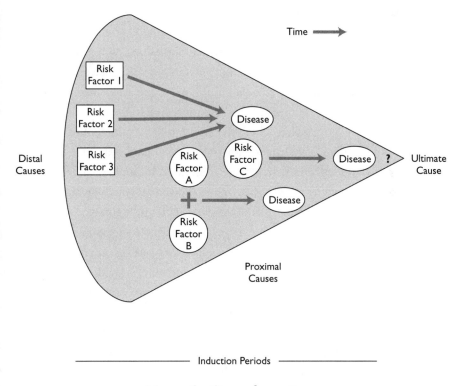

Figure 16.1. Cone of causation.

process. The induction period varies for each causal factor. Some distal environmental factors and minor genetic variations may have induction periods lasting many years, others may last a lifetime, for example, for fetal conditions such as immune system deficiencies, or be intergenerational for epigenetic changes. Proximal causal factors, such as high dose radiation or viral infections, have fairly short induction periods of only a few weeks or months, and ultimate causal factors are virtually instantaneous for risks, such as a chromosome translocation, that immediately influences embryonic development. Another temporal concept, not shown in the figure, is the disease latency period. This follows the induction period and is the time from the onset of disease to when the disease is detected or diagnosed. Screening programs may shorten the latency period but they have no impact on induction times. Importantly, component causes are not fractional and do not add up to 100 percent. They are frequently interactive with each other and, as the figure shows, are a mix of sufficient and necessary causes as described in the previous chapter.

Is identifying the ultimate cause of disease something akin to Zeno's arrow, which after it is halfway to the target has another half to travel, and halfway on still another half, and so on ad infinitum so the arrow never arrives? Is identifying an ultimate cause always one more link in the chain away? Of course, the arrow does arrive, which would seem to be sufficient refutation of Zeno and many causal chains; for example, in cardiovascular disease, teratogenesis and infections have been described by molecular biologists and seem reasonably complete. They have allowed for much greater precision in screening, improved vaccine development, and entirely novel ways of thinking about therapy. As we have seen, some new therapies are based on understanding ultimate causation, such as those using monoclonal antibodies, and are already being offered. But for other conditions, notably for mental diseases, autoimmune diseases, allergies, and some cancers, the cone of causation is far from complete.

The complexity of the causal cone is very varied. The time scale may extend over a lifetime or, as we saw with DES, across generations. Some cardiovascular diseases occurring in older age are thought to have risk factors originating during fetal development. Other diseases have a very short time scale: as soon as the fertilized egg is conceived with an extra chromosome 13, the features of Patau syndrome (severe physical and neurological anomalies) begin to develop in the embryo. The plague bacillus is reported to have produced symptoms in the morning and death by nightfall, but this is somewhat misleading in terms of causality because the antecedent factors that resulted in such a rapid course of disease in some people, while sparing others, includes genetic factors going back to conception. Epigenetic changes are now being observed that once in place continue for several generations. In one recent study, an intense high-fat diet in males resulted in them becoming diabetic. This was not surprising, but what was unexpected is that when these males fathered daughters, they had smaller pancreatic beta cells and more diabetic symptoms. It was found that a gene (*IL13ra2*) had been altered by methylation first in the father, presumably in his sperm, then inherited by the daughter, and this mutation could be passed on to subsequent generations. This experiment was in rats and remains a hypothesis in humans, but it is an entirely plausible explanation for how some diseases may evolve.[8]

The complexity of risk factors incorporated within the causation cone is also very variable. One can imagine a short dose of high-intensity radiation producing damage to the DNA that immediately leads to cellular damage and the rapid onset of a cancer. This is what happened to some of the workers trying to build a containment vessel over the damaged nuclear reactor at Chernobyl, some of whom developed fatal leukemia a few weeks after being exposed. But for most of the diseases that affect us, there are many risk factors, and they are entangled with each other in a seemingly endless variety of ways. Consider asthma: there are likely to be well over 100 genetic variants influencing a wide range of molecular pathways all affecting asthma susceptibility. A very large number of environmental agents have also been found to influence asthma proclivity, some perhaps starting as in utero exposures and many in very early childhood. Further, a large number of asthma "triggers" play on the different susceptibilities and produce asthma symptoms with a wide range of degrees of severity. These are called complex diseases for very good reason.[9]

The language we commonly use to describe causation is often imprecise and hides the true web of causation: for example, smoking does not cause lung cancer; rather, smoking is *a cause* of lung cancer. This reflects several realities: 20 percent of lung cancer occurs in nonsmokers, not all smokers develop cancer, and in some smokers who do develop lung cancer it will not be due to their smoking. Of course, it is always correct to say smoking increases the risk for lung cancer.

A Cone of Curation

Just as the concepts of causality are most often described in terms of disease causation, disease treatment can be considered in a fully analogous way. Although perhaps awkward, it is appropriate to think of causal pathways to recovery or cure from disease, perhaps a web and a cone of curation.[10] Instead of an oncogene turning on and causing disease, it is turned off; rather than a cancer suppressor gene being turned off, it is turned on; proteins are restored instead of being depleted or absent. But the medicine is only the proximal agent in the causal path to recovery; it operates in a network of antecedent factors: does the patient have the genetic constitution to benefit from the therapy, are other drugs being used concomitantly that may enhance or reduce the chance of the medicine being effective, is the patient's diet a factor in causing an interaction with the medicine, and so on. The ultimate curative factors may involve some form of destruction of free radicals, a restoration of immune function, or an end to what is called apoptosis (cell death). An antibiotic can destroy bacteria, but other processes may be needed to bring about full recovery. Likewise, radiation or chemotherapy is only part of a curative chain of events leading to cancer remission.

More precision is also needed in the language of cure to highlight the complexity of the curative process. An effective medicine does not cure a disease; instead, it is *a cure* for the disease. No medicine is able to cure all patients and some patients would have been cured without the medicine. Therapies increase the odds of recovery. More precisely, they decrease the risk of not recovering. (It is conventional in therapy studies to count the worse outcomes.) Chance (perhaps in the form of diagnostic error, the patient wasn't ill with the diagnosed disease), the placebo effect, or natural recovery are all competing explanations that need to be ruled out before a therapy can be reliably documented to have caused recovery. For some surgical, orthopedic, and therapeutic radiology procedures, the causal pathway to recovery may be very short: removal or destruction of the tumor cures the cancer and splinting facilitates the natural healing that "cures" the broken leg. But even this is not as straightforward as it may at first glance seem. Inherent constitutional factors or nuances in surgical technique may result in complete recovery in one patient but not in another treated in ostensibly the same manner.

Risk factors incorporated into cones of causation or curation must be based on valid evidence. Drawing a complex causation cone is not a theoretical exercise that allows any risk factor about which someone has a suspicion to be thrown in. Describing a causation cone is not an excuse for sloppy thinking and speculation. To be a candidate for incorporation into a cone, each risk factor must have met the tests for evidence described throughout this book. Naturally, using stringent evidentiary criteria leaves many holes in the cone, but this accurately reflects incomplete scientific knowledge. Gaps in the cone form the basis for the next set of hypotheses and continuing research.

Concluding Thoughts

This book has focused on how valid evidence is collected to permit judgments about the importance of risk factors in the origins and treatment of disease. It has described how the play of chance always interferes with risk estimation and how determinations of causality are made. I have suggested that individual risk factors may be conceived as interacting within a multifactorial cone of causation. Causation is elusive and studying it the most complex and important task of any scientist interested in the origins and treatment of disease; it is the Holy Grail of medical and public health research. I have argued that treating disease can be viewed conceptually using the same paradigm of causation. The factors bringing about (or causing) a cure include but are not limited to the medicine of interest; there is also a cone of "curation." The closer we come to understanding the ultimate causes of disease, the more effective will be our programs of disease prevention, screening, diagnosis, and treatment. Preventing and treating disease successfully hasn't always needed a complete understanding of how the disease originated but increasingly it will. Uncovering causation is methodologically complex, and, like sailing a boat, there are several ways to do it right and stay on course but a great many more ways to err.

Compared to other sciences, the 1 in 20 criteria for an observation being unlikely to be due to chance, thereby being considered "statistically significant" and so worthy of special attention because it may be causal, is quite liberal. Physicists often use the more conservative sigma 3 rule. Sigma is the symbol for one standard deviation from the mean value of a set of observations and the 1 in 20 or 5 percent rule is approximately based on sigma 2.[11] If we consider the usual bell-shaped curve, sigma 2 on each side of the median value will include 95 percent of the observed data. Observations outside of sigma 2 on each side of the median, under the 5 percent rule, are considered statistically significant.

Sigma 3 has a much more conservative error rate of 1 in 370; moreover, in physics, because only one side of the normal distribution is considered to be able to challenge many physics hypotheses, the error rate is doubled to approximately 1 in 750. In particle physics, an error rate of 1 in 3.5 million (sigma 5) has been used. This is, for example, the test being applied for trying to identify the Higgs boson particle from all the background noise in the particle accelerator experiments. In industrial production, where errors must be maintained at a very low level, the sigma 6 rule is often applied which represents 3.4 errors per million objects. This is actually based on a one-sided sigma of 4.5, which allows for the machines over time incurring increasing error in the precision of the products being manufactured.

These sigma errors apply only to "random error," that is, error occurring in measurement or in experimental design. They do not account for "systematic error", which is described in this book as reporting bias, publication bias, or the other sources of error that are found in the conduct or reporting of experiments. We have discussed elsewhere how these frequently tend to support the reporting of "statistically significant" results that will, in fact, actually be wrong. In light of the downside effects of incorrectly reporting, for example, that a chemical found in the environment (often in miniscule amounts) is associated with an increased risk of cancer, or that a new medicine brings about a cure, a strong case can be made for making nominal tests of significance more stringent. In health research it is usual to use "two-tailed" significance tests. This is so that a drug may be shown to either significantly *improve* a disease outcome or significantly *worsen* it. The usual 1 in 20 rule is called a two-tailed test. A two-tailed error rate of 1 in a 100 (sigma 2.57) is already assumed in health research but has not achieved the routine use it deserves. Perhaps even a two-tailed error rate of sigma 3 (1 in 370) should be adopted to avoid the wasted time and resources that occur in medical science when false leads are being followed.

We should make no mistake that the costs to society are enormous when major clinical trials are launched based on fragile statistical results from animal research or preliminary human data that, while being nominally significant at the 5 percent level, still have an unacceptably high chance of being wrong. Similarly, major public health programs may be launched to remove a suspected cause of cancer, such as electromagnetic fields, from the environment based on statistically unreliable evidence. Given the limited resources available to mount these campaigns this is a zero-sum game; money spent on spurious health campaigns is money not available to tackle much better-documented causes of ill health. A more conservative error rate would require that health researchers conduct more carefully designed and substantially larger, and so more expensive, studies, but this would be well worth the greater certainty that the study result was more likely to be correct.

The public must understand how truly destructive it is to be misled by false claims of harm or of benefit. For example, that nutritional supplements, weight-loss programs, homeopathy, intelligence- and memory-enhancing techniques, and a host of detoxification therapies are beneficial. Or that trace chemicals, electromagnetic radiation, moderate levels of coffee or alcohol, or living near a well-operated nuclear power plant will harm them—all claims made in the absence of reliable supporting evidence and, not infrequently, despite strong negating evidence. There are unintended consequences to these actions: excessive nutrients may actually be harmful (there is reliable evidence that among smokers, beta-carotene supplements appear to increase the risk of lung cancer) or ill-founded claims may distract attention from useful products, and scaremongering detracts from environmental causes that are of genuine concern. Bertrand Russell was only a little harsh when he remarked, "I think the average man would rather face death or torture than think," but "think" we must when faced with a deluge of personal and commercial self-interest that purports to know what is best for our health. Our thoughts must concern the strength of the science underpinning medical and public health policy pronouncements and advertising.

Public health experts too often worry about quite minor risks to health, which diminishes the resources available to manage the major risks. One-fifth of the population of the United States still smokes, which will lead to hundreds of thousands of early and unnecessary deaths. However, much effort has been wasted in trying to control the chemical bisphenol-A (BPA) in food and drink containers when there is no substantial evidence that it causes harm in humans. Moreover, a new strain of an ancient bacterium E. coli, found on a German vegetable farm in the spring of 2011, caused more deaths than any form of genetically modified food, for which there is no evidence of any death or indeed any illness but which is the focus of much angst by some activist groups. Nuclear power generation is without doubt the cleanest, greenest, and safest way to generate electricity on a scale that can substantially lower greenhouse gases, but false alarms about the safety of the industry have undermined sensible government policies, leading in some countries to outright bans on nuclear power generation.[12]

Perhaps most damaging of all is the erosion of the public's trust in science. The public's inability to distinguish reliable sources of knowledge from the hacks and the quacks is the direct result of a desperately inadequate educational system in which even the most rudimentary aspects of how disease risks and disease treatments can be evaluated are never addressed. There is much work to be done. The public should always demand sound evidence to document the claims of causation and successful treatment too often made by purveyors of scam products and scaremongering special interest groups. "Show me the evidence" has to be the watchword of an alert and aware public.

Chapter 1. Risk, Chance, and Causation

1. In this book the term "trial" refers to randomized controlled trials, which are considered to provide the highest level of valid evidence, see chapter 4. "Study" refers to non-randomized study designs. The report showing increased HRT risk was Rossouw JE, Anderson GL, Prentice RL, et al. Risks and benefits of estrogen plus progestin in healthy postmenopausal women: principal results from the Women's Health Initiative randomized controlled trial. *JAMA.* 2002;288(3):321–333. The WHI website provides references to their other studies.
2. The Women's Health Initiative was founded by the United States National Institute of Heart Lung and Blood in 1991 as a series of randomized trials and observational studies to investigate the most common causes of poor health in postmenopausal women. The trials have included more than 160,000 women.
3. Rossouw JE et al. Risks and benefits of estrogen. Op. cit.
4. Bjelakovoc G, Nikolova D, Gluud LL, Simonetti RG, Gluud C. Mortality in randomized trials of antioxidant supplements for primary and secondary prevention. *JAMA.* 2007;297(8):842–857. Overall risk of mortality 1.05 (95%CI 1.02, 1.06).
5. Bønaa KH, Njølstad I, Ueland PM, et al. Homocysteine lowering and cardiovascular events after acute myocardial infarction. *N Engl J Med.* 2006;354(15): 1578–1588.
6. For a more complete reporting of Goldberger's investigations see Terris M. *Goldberger on pellagra.* Terris M, ed. Baton Rouge: Louisiana State University Press; 1964.
7. Goldberger J. The etiology of pellagra: the significance of certain epidemiological observations with respect thereto. *Public Health Rep.* 1914;29(26):1683–1686.
8. Goldberger J. The cause and prevention of pellagra. *Public Health Rep.* 1914;29 (37):2354–2357.

9. Goldberger J, Waring CH, Willets DG. The prevention of pellagra: a test of diet among institutional inmates. *Public Health Rep.* 1915;30(43):3117–3131.

10. Goldberger J, Wheeler GA. The experimental production of pellagra in human subjects by means of diet. *Hygienic Lab Bull.* 1920;120:7–116.

11. See chapter 4 for a discussion of the methodological issues in this study as viewed from a modern perspective.

12. Serious abuse of prisoners involved in medical research resulted, in the early 1970s, in legislation essentially prohibiting their participation except in very special circumstances. A more enlightened view, respecting the autonomy of prisoners, their willingness to assist in medical research, and the protections offered by modern ethics regulation was recently promoted by the Institute of Medicine (*Ethical considerations for research involving prisoners.* Consensus Report; July 12, 2006).

13. Goldberger J. The transmissibility of pellagra: experimental attempts at transmission to the human subject. *Public Health Rep.* 1916;31(46):3159–3173.

14. See Terris M. *Goldberger on pellagra.* Terris M, ed. Baton Rouge: Louisiana State University Press; 1964, for the original papers on these topics.

15. Goldberger J, Tanner WF. A study of the pellagra-preventive action of dried beans, casein, dried milk, and brewers' yeast, with a consideration of the essential preventive factors involved. *Public Health Rep.* 1925;40(2):54–80.

16. Powell K. A life among the viruses. *Yale-Medicine.* 2004 (Fall/Winter):16–17.

17. Palfreyman D, ed. *The Oxford Tutorial*, Oxford, OxCHAPS 2001.

Chapter 2. Chance and Randomness

1. Also given as *Audentes fortuna iuvat* (Fortune favors the daring). The modern English proverb is: "Nothing ventured, nothing gained." The importance of chance in Roman life is exemplified by the many sayings that relate to it: *Fortuna non mutat genus* (Circumstances do not change our origin), *Fortuna obesse nulli contenta est semel* (Fortune is never satisfied with hurting a man just once), *Fortuna vitrea est, tum quum splendet, frangitur* (Fortune is of glass; she glitters just at the moment of breaking), *Fortuna, quum blanditur, fallit* (When fate smiles, it deceives). A complete account of Tyche and Fortuna can be found in Arya DA. The goddess Fortuna in imperial Rome: cult, art, text. PhD diss., University of Texas; 2002.

2. The Victorians even pleaded for the good health of the queen: "*Endue her plenteously with heavenly gifts; grant her in wealth and health long to live; strengthen her that she may vanquish and overcome all her enemies. . . .*" *The Order for Evening Prayer Daily Throughout the Year* in *The Book of Common Prayer.* Oxford: Oxford University Press; 1842. The prayers seemed to have worked in all aspects of Queen Victoria's life but the idea of my ancestor Mary Brunskill, whose prayer book I refer to here, praying every night for Queen Victoria's wealth and the success of her imperial war machine is a little hard to stomach.

3. Eskenazi B, Bracken MB. Bendectin (Debendox) as a risk factor for pyloric stenosis. *Am J Obstet Gynecol.* 1982;144(8):919–924.
4. The role of chance being examined refers to a chance association between a risk factor and a disease, not that the disease was caused by chance.
5. *Obstetrician and Gynaecologist,* Spring 2011.
6. Harr J. *A civil action.* New York: Vintage; 1996. For a more scientific account of the Woburn cluster, see Costas K, Knorr RS, Condon SK. A case control study of childhood leukemia in Woburn, Massachusetts: the relationship between leukemia and exposure to drinking water. *Sci Total Environ.* 2002;300(1–3):23–35.
7. It has proved very difficult to find conclusive evidence for the cause of any cancer cluster. See Boyle P, Walker AM, Alexander FM. Chapter 1. Historical aspects of leukaemia clusters, in Alexander FE, Boyle P, eds. *Methods for investigating localized clustering of disease.* Lyon, France: IARC; 1996.
8. Mary Mallon was an Irish immigrant who cooked for families in New York City. She was forcibly detained for three years and released only after promising not to cook. But she reneged and returned to cooking, infecting additional families, which resulted in more deaths. Mary was again detained, this time for life. Bourdain A. *Typhoid Mary.* New York: Bloomsbury Press; 2001; Leavitt JW. *Typhoid Mary: captive to the public's health.* Boston: Beacon Press; 1996.
9. The classic book on the early history of the AIDs epidemic continues to be Shilts R. *And the band played on: politics, people and the AIDS epidemic.* New York: St. Martin's Press; 1987.
10. Rothman KJ. *Modern epidemiology.* 1st ed. Boston: Little, Brown; 1986:78.
11. There are several variations of Dawkins's quote on this theme. This one is from *Forbes* magazine, 1999.

Chapter 3. Risk

1. That evening, July 21, 2010, we later learned, had seen half a dozen tornadoes in southern Maine with major tree damage and reports of water spouts some 30 miles east of Dix Harbor. It seems that we were caught in a local microburst, on the edge of some very severe weather. Tornadoes were reported from Connecticut and severe weather conditions in Pennsylvania and New Jersey. I could never get a good look at the wind speed indicator, which was in the cockpit, but judge we were in severe gale conditions at the height of the storm.
2. A more recent derivation appears to be from the nineteenth-century French *risqué*; although in seventeenth-century Germany *rysigo* became a term to imply the now very familiar notion of risk associated with business ventures.
3. Relative risk is the most commonly used statistic for calculating risk. It is derived from prospectively designed studies, including clinical trials and contrasts the risk of disease in a population exposed to a risk factor compared to the risk

of disease in an unexposed population. Chapter 8 provides the formula. Another statistic, the odds ratio, is widely used in medical research, and it is an estimation of relative risk derived from *retrospective* studies where the risks in exposed and unexposed subjects cannot be directly calculated, the odds ratio is a reasonably precise estimate of relative risk when the prevalence of the disease in the population is < 10 percent (see chapter 8 for how it is calculated). However, the odds ratio can also overestimate the relative risk in important ways. See Sinclair JC, Bracken MB. Clinically useful measures of effect in binary analyses of randomized trials. *J Clin Epidemiol.* 1994;47(8):881–889; and Bracken MB, Sinclair JC. When can odds ratios mislead? Avoidable systematic error in estimating treatment effect must not be tolerated. *BMJ.* 1998;317(7166):1156.

4. Wynder EL, Graham EA. Tobacco smoking as a possible etiologic factor in bronchogenic carcinoma: a study of six hundred and eighty-four proved cases. *JAMA.* 1950;143(4):329–336; Doll R, Hill AB. Smoking and carcinoma of the lung: preliminary report. *Br Med J.* 1950;2(4682):739–748. The history of the early research into smoking and lung cancer has been well summarized by Colin White. White C. Research on smoking and lung cancer: a landmark in the history of chronic disease epidemiology. *Yale J Biol Med.* 1990;63(1):29–46.

5. Cornfield J, Haenzel W, Hammond EC, Lilienfeld AM, Shimkin MB, Wynder EL. Smoking and lung cancer: recent evidence and a discussion of some questions. *J Natl Cancer Inst.* 1959;22(1):173–203.

6. Poole C. On the origin of risk relativism. *Epidemiology.* 2010;21(1):3–9.

7. The occurrence of new disease is called "incidence" by epidemiologists. The measure of existing disease is "prevalence." For example, the incidence of new cases of diabetes in the United States in 2010 for people 20 years and older was 1.9 million and the prevalence was 25.6 million cases or 11.3 percent of the population. This translates into an annual risk of developing diabetes of about 1 percent per year. For birth defects, however, the rate of new cases is also called prevalence because many birth defects are spontaneously aborted before birth.

8. As of this writing, the actual genetic variation that may account for the very high twinning rate in Cândido Godói has not been revealed. Natural twinning rates, of fraternal twins, vary across the world but usually not by a factor of 10, indicating that this is most unlikely to be a chance increase in risk. In southwest Nigeria, among the Yoruba, the twinning rate is four to five times the rate in Europe, and consumption of yams that have a high level of estrogen-like compounds has been suggested as the risk factor. However, yams are consumed throughout Africa, where twinning rates are not consistently high, which suggests a local genetic factor may also play a role in the high twinning rate, particularly if there is some inbreeding within the tribal areas. In contrast to fraternal (dizygotic) twins, the rate of identical (monozygotic twin birth) is remarkably constant across populations, at about 0.5 percent of all births.

9. Bracken MB. Incidence and aetiology of hydatidiform mole: an epidemiological review. *Br J Obstet Gynaecol.* 1987;94(12):1123–1135; Lurain JR. Gestational trophoblastic diseases 1: epidemiology, pathology, clinical presentation and diagnosis of gestational trophoblastic disease, and management of hydatidiform mole. *Am J Obstet Gynecol.* 2010;203(6):531–539.

10. Koren G, Pastuszak A, Ito S. Drugs in pregnancy. *New Engl J Med.* 1998; 338(16):1128–1137; The Drug Safety Society website. Taking Thalidomide during pregnancy and breastfeeding. http://thedrugsafety.com/thalidomide/. Accessed April 25, 2012. Widespread use of thalidomide was prevented in the United States by Dr. Frances Kelsey, an FDA safety officer, who became suspicious that the drug's safety record had not been fully revealed. Her work saved countless newborns from serious malformations, for which in 1962 she was awarded the President's Award for Distinguished Federal Civilian Service by President Kennedy. Following this incident, the Food and Drug Administration made substantial improvements to the manner in which drugs used in pregnancy are regulated.

11. Calculated by 1 − relative risk × 100%.

12. Goldacre B. Bad Science: Do 600 unwanted pregnancies really make an exceptional story? Media claims about contraceptive implant "failure" don't put figures into context. *Guardian.* http://www.guardian.co.uk/commentisfree/2011/jan/08/bad-science-implant-pregnancies. Published January 7, 2011. Accessed April 25, 2012.

13. Loke YK, Kwok CS, Singh S. Comparative cardiovascular effects of thiazolidinediones: a systematic review and meta-analysis of observational studies. *BMJ.* 2011;342:d1309.

14. National Academy of Sciences. *Health risks from dioxin and related compounds: evaluation of the EPA reassessment.* Washington, DC: National Academies Press; 2006.

15. Montori VM, Jaeschke R, Schünemann HJ, et al. Users' guide to detecting misleading claims in clinical research reports. *BMJ.* 2004;329(7474):1093–1096.

Chapter 4. Randomization and Clinical Trials

1. Bias refers to systematic errors in the design, conduct, or analysis of a study that lead to inaccurate findings.

2. John Ioannidis has written extensively and thoughtfully on this topic. See, for example, Ioannidis J. Why most published research findings are false. *PLoS Med.* 2005;2(8):e124.; Ioannidis JPA. Why most discovered true associations are inflated. *Epidemiology.* 2008;19(5):640–648; Ioannidis JPA. Sequential discovery, thinking versus dredging, and shrink or sink (commentary). *Epidemiology.* 2008;19(5):657–658; Young NS, Ioannides JP, Al-Ubaydli O. Why current publication practices may distort science? *PLoS Med.* 2008;5(10):e201.

3. For more about Lind's medical investigations, see Tröhler U. James Lind and the evaluation of clinical practice. *JLL Bulletin: Commentaries on the history of treatment evaluation*. James Lind Library (www.jameslindlibrary.org); 2003. Accessed April 26, 2012.

4. Soranus, of Ephesus. *Gynaecology*. Temkin O, trans. Baltimore: Johns Hopkins University Press; 1956.

5. In Daniel, writing circa 606 BCE, the king of Judah took charge of four healthy and intelligent children whom he wanted to feed on meat and wine. One child was Daniel who preferred "pulse" (legumes) and water. He persuaded the overseeing eunuch to feed them this for ten days and then to compare their "countenances" with children fed the king's diet. "And at the end of ten days their countenances appeared fairer and fatter in flesh than all the children which did eat the portion of the king's meat" (Daniel 1:15).

6. Lowenstein PR, Castro MG. Uncertainty in the translation of preclinical experiments to clinical trials: why do most phase III clinical trials fail? *Curr Gene Ther.* 2009;9(5):368–374.

7. Many therapies for treating tuberculosis involved repeatedly collapsing the lung using a variety of techniques, such as inserting porcelain balls or breaking several ribs and pushing them into the thorax.

8. Sir Austin Bradford Hill, one of the most formidable medical scientists of the twentieth century, made numerous contributions to epidemiology, medical statistics, and understanding the difficulty of ascribing causality to observed associations, and he proposed a construct for doing so that is still widely used to this day (chapter 15).

9. A Medical Research Council Investigation. Streptomycin treatment of pulmonary tuberculosis. *Br Med J.* 1948;2(4582):769–782. The main outcome "considerable improvement" had a relative risk of 5.6 (95%CI 1.49, 16.6) and the number needed to treat was 3 (95%CI 2, 4), that is, for every 3 treated patients one would show considerable improvement due to the streptomycin; death was protected by streptomycin RR = 0.73 (95%CI 0.23, 0.90), NNH for bed rest was 5 (95%CI 3, 18). These statistical results, calculated by the author, demonstrate a strong benefit of therapy that would still be considered impressive using modern standards of data reporting.

10. Sir Richard Peto is an eminent Oxford epidemiologist who has made many contributions to the design of RCTs, the epidemiology of smoking-related disease, meta-analysis, and medical statistics. His first of several influential papers on the design of randomized trials were: Peto R, Pike MC, Armitage P, et al. Design and analysis of randomized clinical trials requiring prolonged observation of each patient. I. Introduction and design. *Br J Cancer.* 1976;34(6):585–612, and Peto R, Pike MC, Armitage P, et al. Design and analysis of randomized clinical trials requiring prolonged observation of each patient. II. Analysis and examples. *Br J Cancer.* 1977;35(1):1–39.

11. Minimization is a widely used strategy in large trials that has the advantage of preserving a balance in important co-variables while preserving some element of pure

randomization. During the minimization process, the patient's information on the co-variables of interest are computed and compared to the frequency of the same co-variables of subjects already enrolled into the study. If these are assessed as being uneven between the treatment groups, the randomization process is weighted to increase the probability of randomizing the new patient so as to redress the lack of balance on the co-variates. This determinative probability is never 100 percent so that some element of chance is maintained in the allocation to treatment process.

12. One of the most famous RCTs of a surgical intervention was a comparison of breast cancer surgery where the dominant surgical procedure of the time, radical mastectomy, was compared to a much more conservative procedure called lumpectomy. This trial, which many thought could never be done because it exposed women to not being adequately treated by the widely accepted radical surgery, showed the same survival rates from both procedures and led to widespread adoption of lumpectomy. Fisher B, Bauer M, Margolese R, et al. Five-year results of a randomized clinical trial comparing total mastectomy and segmental mastectomy with or without radiation in the treatment of breast cancer. *N Engl J Med.* 1985;312(11):665–673.

13. Modern trials are now routinely monitored by data safety monitoring boards that also try to examine trends in the accumulating trial data so as to ensure that there are no unanticipated increases in complications, or that the trial has achieved its objectives earlier than expected, using masked data from equally masked data analysts. It is necessary to be very careful that, with all the masking, one does not confuse what the actual assignment groups really are. At least one trial was published reversing the treatment and control groups that was only discovered when the data were submitted for meta-analysis.

14. Chalmers T. Randomize the first patient. *N Engl J Med.* 1977;296(2):107. Tom Chalmers once confided in me that he knew of only four examples where this had actually been done, and he was responsible for all of them.

15. Spencer DD, Robbins RJ, Naftolin F, et al. Unilateral transplantation of human fetal mesencephalic tissue into the caudate nucleus of patients with Parkinson's disease. *N Engl J Med.* 1992;327(22):1541–1548.

16. Hill KP, Ross JS, Egilman DS, Krumholz HM. The ADVANTAGE seeding trial: a review of internal documents. *Ann Intern Med.* 2008;149(4):251–258.

Chapter 5. More Trials and Some Tribulations

1. Edition critique par L. Retat. Paris, CNRS Editions; 1992.

2. Horbar JD, Carpenter JH, Buzas J, et al. Collaborative quality improvement to promote evidence based surfactant for preterm infants: a cluster randomised trial. *BMJ.* 2004;329(7473):1004.

3. The most comprehensive text on crossover trials is Senn S. *Cross-over trials in clinical research.* 2nd ed. Chichester, UK: John Wiley; 2002.

4. Zhang G, Hou R, Zhou H, et al. Improved sedation for dental extraction by using video eyewear in conjunction with nitrous oxide: a randomized controlled, cross-over clinical trial. *Oral Surg Oral Med Oral Pathol Oral Radiol Endod.* 2011 Apr 20. (Epub ahead of print.)

5. Peto R, Baigent C. Trials: the next 50 years: large scale randomised evidence of moderate benefits. *BMJ.* 1998;317(7167):1170–1171.

6. Yusuf S, Collins R, Peto R. Why do we need some large, simple randomized trials? *Stat Med.* 1984;3(4):409–422.

7. Peto R, Baigent C. Trials: the next 50 years. Op. cit.

8. CAST: randomised placebo-controlled trial of early aspirin use in 20,000 patients with acute ischaemic stroke. CAST (Chinese Acute Stroke Trial) Collaborative Group. *Lancet.* 1997;349(9066):1641–1649.

9. Edwards P, Arango M, Balica L, et al. and CRASH trial collaborators. Final results of MRC CRASH, a randomised placebo-controlled trial of intravenous corticosteroid in adults with head injury-outcomes at 6 months. *Lancet.* 2005;365(9475): 1957–1959.

10. Blot WJ, Li JY, Taylor PR, et al. Nutrition intervention trials in Linxian, China: supplementation with specific vitamin/mineral combinations, cancer incidence, and disease-specific mortality in the general population. *J Natl Cancer Inst.* 1993;85(18):1483–1492.

11. Bracken MB, Shepard MJ, Collins WF, et al. A randomized, controlled trial of methylprednisolone or naloxone in the treatment of acute spinal-cord injury: results of the Second National Acute Spinal Cord Injury Study. *N Engl J Med.* 1990;322(20):1405–1411.

12. Baigent C, Collins R, Appleby P, Parish S, Sleight P, Peto R. ISIS-2: 10 year survival among patients with suspected acute myocardial infarction in randomised comparison of intravenous streptokinase, oral aspirin, both, or neither. The ISIS2 (Second International Study of Infarct Survival) Collaborative Group. *BMJ.* 1998;316(7141):1337–1343.

13. Taves DR. Minimization: a new method of assigning patients to treatment and control groups. *Clin Pharmacol Ther.* 1974;15(5):443–453.

14. Bracken MB, Shepard MJ, Collins WF, et al. A randomized, controlled trial of methylprednisolone or naloxene. Op. cit.

15. See note 9, above, for the CRASH trial and note 11 for the spinal injury trial citations. Roberts I, Prieto-Merino D, Shakur H, Chalmers I, Nicholl J. Effect of consent rituals on mortality in emergency care research. *Lancet.* 2011;377(9771): 1071–1072. This paper has the full reference to the original tranexamic acid trial (CRASH-2 trial collaborators, Shakur H, Roberts I, et al. Effects of tranexamic acid on death, vascular occlusive events, and blood transfusion in trauma patients with significant haemorrhage (CRASH-2): a randomised, placebo-controlled trial. *Lancet.* 2010;376(9734):23–32. For an examination of the paradox that demands

different ethical standards in and outside trials, see Chalmers I. Regulation of therapeutic research is compromising the interests of patients. *Int J Pharm Med.* 2007;21(6):395–404.

16. Lawlor DA, Nelson SM. Effect of age on decisions about the number of embryos to transfer in assisted conception: a prospective study. *Lancet.* 2012;379(9815):521–527.

17. Schuster B. Police lineups: making eyewitness identification more reliable. *NIJ Journal.* 2007; No. 258.

Chapter 6. Harm

1. Common complications may be detected in the randomized trials done to show the effectiveness of a therapy and described in earlier chapters; however, very few trials are large enough to detect rare side effects, for example, those that occur in 1 per 1,000 exposed patients but which are important to detect when tens of thousands or even millions of people may be exposed to the drug or chemical.

2. Validity (reduced bias) and precision are two of the key general considerations in designing an observational study, and they often compete for attention. Large studies may be designed which do not pay sufficient attention to collecting unbiased data, whereas smaller studies may pay more attention to these details but lack precision. It is always preferred to enhance validity over precision; an invalid study serves no purpose and may lead to incorrect conclusions. The precision of small but valid studies can be improved in meta-analysis (chapter 13).

3. This calculation assumes a 3 per 100,000 incidence of glioma, and 30 percent of the population of interest uses cell phones.

4. There are many types of bias. In the 1970s a conference of epidemiologists on Bermuda identified 56 types of bias in the epidemiological literature. One cannot help but surmise that if the meeting had gone on several days longer, imagination and the holiday atmosphere might have suggested many more. Indeed, most recently a science mapping analysis found 235 biases used in biomedical research. Sackett DL. Bias in analytic research. *J Chronic Dis.* 1979;32(1–2):51–63; Chavalarias D, Ioannidis JP. Science mapping analysis characterizes 235 biases in biomedical research. *J Clin Epidemiol.* 2010;63(11):1205–1215.

5. Bar-Oz B, Einarson T, Einarson A, et al. Paroxetine and congenital malformations: meta-analysis and consideration of potential confounding factors. *Clin Ther.* 2007;29(5):918–926.

6. Wogelius P, Nørgaard M, Gislum M, et al. Maternal use of selective serotonin reuptake inhibitors and risk of congenital malformations. *Epidemiology.* 2006; 17(6):701–704.

7. Wertheimer N, Leeper E. Electrical wiring configurations and childhood cancer. *Am J Epidemiol.* 1979;109(3):273–284.

8. Kheifets L, Monroe J, Vergara X, Mezei G, Afifi AA. Occupational electro-magnetic fields and leukemia and brain cancer: an update of two meta-analyses. *J Occup Environ Med.* 2008;50(6):677–688.

9. Melbye M, Wohlfahrt J, Olsen JH, et al. Induced abortion and the risk of breast cancer. *N Engl J Med.* 1997;336(2):81–85.

10. MacMahon B, Yen S, Trichopoulos D, Warren K, Nardi G. Coffee and cancer of the pancreas. *N Engl J Med.* 1981;304(11):630–633.

11. When many associations are examined in a statistical analysis, the traditional p-value (typically $p < 0.05$ α-level) is invalid. Statistical tests evaluate the probability that an observation is due to chance, for example, assuming a 1 per 20 likelihood that the observation is due to chance is an appropriate criterion (some scientists prefer a criterion of 1 per 100). However, under the 1 per 20 criterion, if 100 associations are examined in a study (say from comparing 5 drug exposures in pregnancy with 20 different congenital malformations), then 5 associations will be observed at the $p < 0.05$ level merely by chance. Falsely attributing these as being statistically significant associations is an example of what is called type 1 error. A simple correction for multiple comparison bias, attributed to the Italian statistician Bonferroni, is to use a new p-value calculated by 0.05/number associations examined. In the example above, the corrected p-value becomes 0.05/100 = 0.0005. The 0.05 significance level is not a limit that precludes further study of "nonsignificant" findings but rather a convention for identifying studies that are of particular interest and merit further research. In the search for causality, there has not been a causal association that does not also meet the standards of statistical significance. But this does not mean that all nonsignificant associations should be ignored. Nonsignificant associations in early research may become statistically significant when better studies are conducted, although in practice many do not.

12. Gent JF, Triche EW, Holford TR, et al. Association of low-level ozone and fine particles with respiratory symptoms in children with asthma. *JAMA.* 2003;290(14):1859–1867.

13. Johansen D, Friis K, Skovenborg E, Grønbaek M. Food buying habits of people who buy wine or beer: cross sectional study. *BMJ.* 2006;332(7540):519–522.

14. There was evidence that conductors were less overweight than drivers at the time they started their jobs, but Morris and colleagues were able to correct for this in making their calculations of risk. There is no evidence that they were more likely to have early signs of heart disease. Morris JN, Heady JA, Raffle PA, Roberts CG, Parks JW. Coronary heart-disease and physical activity of work. *Lancet.* 1953;265(6795):1053–1057; contd., and Morris JN, Heady JA, Raffle PA, Roberts CG, Parks JW. Coronary heart-disease and physical activity of work. *Lancet.* 1953;265(6796):1111–1120; concl. For a general discussion, see Paffenbarger RS Jr, Blair SN, Lee IM. A history of physical activity, cardiovascular health and longevity: the scientific contributions of Jeremy N Morris, DSc, DPH, FRCP. *Int J Epidemiol.* 2001;30(5):1184–1192.

15. Risnes KR, Belanger K, Murk W, Bracken MB. Antibiotic exposure by 6 months and asthma and allergy at 6 years: Findings in a cohort of 1,401 US children. *Am J Epidemiol.* 2011;173(3):310–318; Murk W, Risnes KR, Bracken MB. Prenatal or early-life exposure to antibiotics and risk of childhood asthma: a systematic review. *Pediatrics.* 2011;127(6):1125–1138.
16. Bracken MB. *Perinatal Epidemiology.* New York: Oxford University Press; 1984:424, 426.
17. Botto LD, Lin AE, Riehle-Colarusso T, Malik S, Correa A. National Birth Defects Prevention Study: seeking causes: classifying and evaluating congenital heart defects in etiologic studies. *Birth Defects Res A Clin Mol Teratol.* 2007;79(10):714–727.
18. Höfer T, Przyrembel H, Verleger S. New evidence for the theory of the stork. *Paediatr Perinat Epidemiol.* 2004;18(1):88–92.
19. Goldacre B. Press bandwagon on antidepressants makes for depressing read. *Guardian.* http://www.guardian.co.uk/science/2011/apr/09/ben-goldacre-bad-science-antidepressants. Published April 8, 2011. Accessed April 23, 2012.
20. Cook DL. The Hawthorne effect in educational research. *Phi Delta Kappan.* 1962;44(3):116–122.

Chapter 7. Screening, Diagnosis, and Prognosis

1. The American College of Obstetricians and Gynecologists provides an example of a breast self-examination guideline. The American College of Obstetricians and Gynecologists website. *Breast self-exam.* http://www.acog.org/~/media/For%20 Patients/faq145.pdf?dmc=1&ts=20120425T1447577880. Accessed April 23, 2012.
2. Thomas DB, Gao DL, Ray RM, et al. Randomized trial of breast self-examination in Shanghai: final results. *J Natl Cancer Inst.* 2002;94(19):1445–1457. I have calculated from this trial the likelihood ratio of detecting an invasive in situ cancer as 0.98; the pretest probability of detecting the cancer as 0.007; the posttest probability is the same, 0.007, showing absolutely no benefit.
3. Gøtzsche PC, Nielsen M. Screening for breast cancer with mammography. *Cochrane Database Syst Rev.* 2011;(1):CD001877.
4. Moss SM, Cuckle H, Evans A, Johns L, Waller M, Bobrow L; Trial Management Group. Effect of mammographic screening from age 40 years on breast cancer mortality at 10 years' follow-up: a randomised controlled trial. *Lancet.* 2006;368(9552):2053–2060; Johns LE, Moss SM; Age Trial Management Group. False-positive results in the randomized controlled trial of mammographic screening from age 40 ("Age" trial). *Cancer Epidemiol Biomarkers Prev.* 2010;19(11):2758–2764.
5. Djulbegovic M, Beyth RJ, Neuberger MM, et al. Screening for prostate cancer: systematic review and meta-analysis of randomized controlled trials. *BMJ.* 2010;341:c4543; Kilpeläinen TP, Tammela TL, Määttänen L, et al. False-positive screening results in the Finnish prostate cancer screening trial. *Br J Cancer.*

2010;102(3):469–474; Esserman L, Shieh Y, Thompson I. Rethinking screening for breast cancer and prostate cancer. *JAMA.* 2009;302(15):1685–1692.

6. United States Preventive Services Task Force (USPSTF) website. Screening for prostate cancer: U.S. Preventive Services Task Force Recommendation Statement. http://www.uspreventiveservicestaskforce.org/uspstf12/prostate/draftrecprostate.htm. Accessed April 24, 2012.

7. Andriole GL, Crawford ED, Grubb RL 3rd, et al.; and PLCO Project Team. Mortality results from a randomized prostate-cancer screening trial. *N Engl J Med.* 2009;360(13):1310–1319; Schröder FH, Hugosson J, Roobol MJ, et al; and ERSPC Investigators. Screening and prostate-cancer mortality in a randomized European study. *N Engl J Med.* 2009;360(13):1320–1328.

8. Medeiros LR, Rosa DD, da Rosa MI, Bozzetti MC. Accuracy of CA 125 in the diagnosis of ovarian tumors: a quantitative systematic review. *Eur J Obstet Gynecol Reprod Biol.* 2009;142(2):99–105; Rustin GJ, Nelstrop AE, Tuxen MK, Lambert HE. Defining progression of ovarian carcinoma during follow-up according to CA 125: a North Thames Ovary Group Study. *Ann Oncol.* 1996;7(4):361–364; Karam AK, Karlan BY. Ovarian cancer: the duplicity of CA-125 measurement. *Nat Rev Clin Oncol.* 2010;7(6):335–339; Anderson GL. Ovarian cancer biomarker screening: still too early to tell. *Womens Health (Lond Engl).* 2010;6(4):487–490.

9. Two examples of work trying to identify useful prognostic biomarkers are Gould Rothberg BE, Bracken MB. E-cadherin immunohistochemical expression as a prognostic factor in infiltrating ductal carcinoma of the breast: a systematic review and meta-analysis. *Breast Cancer Res Treat.* 2006;100(2):139–148; and Gould Rothberg BE, Bracken MB, Rimm DL. Tissue biomarkers for prognosis in cutaneous melanoma: a systematic review and meta-analysis. *J Natl Cancer Inst.* 2009;101(7):452–474.

10. Feinstein AR, Sosin DM, Wells CK. The Will Rogers phenomenon: stage migration and new diagnostic techniques as a source of misleading statistics for survival in cancer. *N Engl J Med.* 1985;312(25):1604–1608.

11. The science of screening invokes the terms "sensitivity" and "specificity." Higher sensitivity refers to the test detecting more disease correctly, and the higher specificity refers to correctly detecting people without the disease. Optimizing sensitivity and specificity is done using Receiver Operating Curve analysis. A major text describing this is Sackett D, Haynes RB, Guyatt GH, Tugwell P. *Clinical epidemiology: a basic science for clinical medicine.* 2nd ed. Boston: Little, Brown; 1991.

Chapter 8. A Statistical Sojourn

1. Venn (1866) introduced concepts of statistical significance. A historical perspective is in Hurlbert SH, Lombardi CM. Final collapse of the Neyman-Pearson decision theoretic framework and rise of the neoFisherian. *Ann Zool Fennici.* 2009;46(5):311–349.

2. Bonferroni CE. *Teoria statistica delle classi e calcolo delle probabilita.* Volume in onore di Riccardo Dalla Volta. Universitá di Firenze. 1937:1–62.

3. "Absence of evidence is not evidence of absence" is widely attributed to Carl Sagan, who also brought us: "If you want to make apple pie from scratch, you must first create the universe," but it most likely originated with fellow astronomer Martin Rees.

4. Bolles RC. The difference between statistical hypotheses and scientific hypotheses. *Psychol Rep.* 1962;11:639–645.

5. Ioannidis JP. Why most published research findings are false. *PLoS Med.* 2005;2(8):e124.

6. Clinical trials are actually monitored in this fashion; the risk estimate (or sometimes the p-value) is tracked as patients enter the trial, and when it crosses a "significance threshold" the trial is stopped. This "stopping rule" threshold is set at a conservative level so that the trial is not stopped prematurely.

7. Hanley JA, Lippman-Hand A. If nothing goes wrong, is everything all right? Interpreting zero numerators. *JAMA.* 1983;249(13):1743–1745.

8. Thomas Bayes (1702–1761) was an English clergyman and amateur mathematician. Probability tests in the Bayes paradigm use extant knowledge to develop a "prior probability" which is multiplied by the likelihood derived from the study data to derive a "posterior probability." Note the similarity of this approach to what is described in the text for screening test data.

9. Sinclair JC, Bracken MB. Clinically useful measures of effect in binary analyses of randomized trials. *J Clin Epidemiol.* 1994;47(8):881–889.

10. Naylor CD, Chen E, Strauss B. Measured enthusiasm: does the method of reporting trial results alter perceptions of therapeutic effectiveness? *Ann Intern Med.* 1992;117(11):916–921. The data used here are from Bracken MB. Chapter 2: Statistical methods for analysis of effects of treatment in overviews of randomized trials. In Sinclair JC, Bracken MB. *Effective care of the newborn infant.* Oxford: Oxford University Press; 1992:14.

11. Thomas DB, Gao DL, Ray RM, et al. Randomized trial of breast self-examination in Shanghai: final results. *J Natl Cancer Inst.* 2002;94(19):1445–1457.

12. The likelihood ratio, which is the principal statistic used for assessing screening and diagnostic tests, is calculated by (sensitivity/1 − specificity) and interpreted as: given a positive test result, the likelihood that a patient comes from a disease population versus coming from a non-disease population. Likelihood ratios of > 10 or < 0.1 are said to provide "convincing" evidence of screening or diagnostic test results; ratios of > 5 or < 0.2 provide "strong" evidence.

"Sensitivity" is the proportion of true positive cases identified, and "specificity" is the proportion of true negative cases identified.

Chapter 9. Disease Clusters

1. I cannot be certain that these are not "fake" memories, induced by decades of family lore and war stories.

2. More details of the Minamata cluster are at Allchin D. *The poisoning of Minamata*. University of Minnesota, SHiPS Resource Center website. www1.umn.edu/ships/ethics/minamata.htm. Accessed April 26, 2012.

3. The problem became a major public health concern due to the large number of people in Connecticut employed by Pratt and Whitney and the state commissioner of health appointed a Scientific Advisory Committee, which I chaired, to advise him about the progress of the research, conducted by the University of Pittsburgh.

4. Marsh GM, Buchanich JM, Youk AO, et al. Long-term health experience of jet engine manufacturing workers: I. Mortality from central nervous system neoplasms. *J Occup Environ Med.* 2008;50(10):1099–1116; Marsh GM, Buchanich JM, Youk AO, et al. Long-term health experience of jet engine manufacturing workers: III. Incidence of malignant central nervous system neoplasms. *Neuroepidemiology.* 2010;35(2):123–141.

5. Alexander FE, Boyle P, eds. *Methods for investigating localized clustering of disease*. IARC Scientific Publications No. 135. Lyon, France: IARC; 1996.

6. Steere AC, Malawista SE, Snydman DR, et al. Lyme arthritis: an epidemic of oligoarticular arthritis in children and adults in three Connecticut communities. *Arthritis Rheum.* 1977;20(1):7–17.

7. Steere AC, Malawista SE, Hardin JA, Ruddy S, Askenase W, Andiman WA. Erythema chronicum migrans and Lyme arthritis: the enlarging clinical spectrum. *Ann Intern Med.* 1977;86(6):685–698; Steere AC, Broderick TF, Malawista SE. Erythema chronicum migrans and Lyme arthritis: epidemiologic evidence for a tick vector. *Am J Epidemiol.* 1978;108(4):312–321.

8. A vaccine (LYMErix) with 78 percent effectiveness was developed by Smith Kline Beecham and received FDA approval in 1999. Concerns about side effects, especially in people who already had arthritis or heart conditions, and also poor sales, led to withdrawal of the vaccine by the company in 2002. A continuing controversy about Lyme disease concerns what Dr. Steere called "junk drawer diagnosis." This refers to a Lyme disease diagnosis being incorrectly ascribed to other conditions with similar signs and symptoms that are then treated inappropriately with very large doses of antibiotics.

Chapter 10. Genetics and the Genome

Excerpt from "This Be The Verse" from *The Complete Poems of Philip Larkin* by Philip Larkin, edited by Archie Burnett. Copyright © 2012 by The Estate of Philip Larkin. Introduction copyright © 2012 by Archie Burnett. Published by Farrar, Straus and Giroux LLC and Faber and Faber Ltd.

1. The human genome was first sequenced and simultaneously published by two groups, a public university-based project and another by Celera, a private company. It is widely believed that the competition this engendered facilitated the timely completion of the project. Lander ES, Linton LM, Birren B, et al. and

International Human Genome Sequencing Consortium. Initial sequencing and analysis of the human genome. *Nature.* 2001;409(6822):860–921.

2. International HapMap Consortium. A haplotype map of the human genome. *Nature.* 2005;437(7063):1299–1320.

3. Bracken MB, DeWan A, Hoh J. Genome wide association studies. In Rebbeck TR, Ambrosone CA, Shields PG, eds. *Molecular epidemiology: applications in cancer and other human diseases.* New York: Informa Healthcare USA; 2008.

4. Klein RJ, Zeiss C, Chew EY, et al. Complement factor H polymorphism in age-related macular degeneration. *Science.* 2005;308(5720):385–389; Dewan A, Liu M, Hartman S, et al. HTRA1 promoter polymorphism in wet age-related macular degeneration. *Science.* 2006;314(5801):989–992.

5. It was estimated in 2011 by bioinformatics experts at Yale University that one complete human genome needed 500 GB of storage and 3,000 processing hours of CPU time. The respective units for an exome were 10 GB and 60 hours.

6. Choi M, Scholl UI, Ji W, et al. Genetic diagnosis by whole exome capture and massively parallel DNA sequencing. *Proc Natl Acad Sci USA.* 2009;106(45): 19096–19101.

7. Wei X, Walia V, Lin JC, et al. Exome sequencing identifies GRIN2A as frequently mutated in melanoma. *Nat Genet.* 2011;43(5):442–446.

8. Vissers LE, de Ligt J, Gilissen C, et al. A de novo paradigm for mental retardation. *Nat Genet.* 2010;42(12):1109–1112.

9. Walsh KM, Bracken MB. Copy number variation in the dosage-sensitive 16p11.2 interval accounts for only a small proportion of autism incidence: a systematic review and meta-analysis. *Genet Med.* 2011;13(5):377–384.

10. Bracken MB. Cotinine and spontaneous abortion: might variations in metabolism play a role? *Epidemiology.* 2006;17(5):492–494; Grosso LM, Bracken MB. Caffeine metabolism, genetics, and perinatal outcomes: a review of exposure assessment considerations during pregnancy. *Ann Epidemiol.* 2005;15(6):460–466; Cornelis MC, Monda KL, Yu K, et al. Genome-wide meta-analysis identifies regions on 7p21 (AHR) and 15q24 (CYP1A2) as determinants of habitual caffeine consumption. *PLoS Genet.* 2011;7(4):e1002033.

11. Johnson EO, Chen LS, Breslau N, et al. Peer smoking and the nicotinic receptor genes: an examination of genetic and environmental risks for nicotine dependence. *Addiction.* 2010;105(11):2014–2022.

12. Cantonwine D, Hu H, Téllez-Rojo MM, et al. HFE gene variants modify the association between maternal lead burden and infant birthweight: a prospective birth cohort study in Mexico City, Mexico. *Environ Health.* 2010;9:43.

13. De Moor MH, Spector TD, Cherkas LF, et al. Genome-wide linkage scan for athlete status in 700 British female DZ twin pairs. *Twin Res Hum Genet.* 2007; 10(6):812–820.

14. Bartels M, Saviouk V, de Moor MH, et al. Heritability and genome-wide linkage scan of subjective happiness. *Twin Res Hum Genet.* 2010;13(2):135–142.

15. Wang X, Shaffer JR, Weyant RJ, et al. Genes and their effects on dental caries may differ between primary and permanent dentitions. *Caries Res.* 2010;44(3):277–84.

16. Nature Insight: Epigenetics. *Nature.* 2007;447(7143):396–440; Halušková J. Epigenetic studies in human diseases. *Folia Biol (Praha).* 2010;56(3):83–96.

17. Karberg S. Switching on epigenetic therapy. *Cell.* 2009;139(6):1029–1031; Egger G, Liang G, Aparicio A, Jones PA. Epigenetics in human disease and prospects for epigenetic therapy. *Nature.* 2004;429(6990):457–463.

18. Garfield AS, Cowley M, Smith FM, et al. Distinct physiological and behavioural functions for parental alleles of imprinted *Grb10. Nature.* 2011;469(7331): 534–538.

19. Hines LM, Stampfer MJ, Ma J, et al. Genetic variation in alcohol dehydrogenase and the beneficial effect of moderate alcohol consumption on myocardial infarction. *N Engl J Med.* 2001;344(8):549–555. For a general review of Mendelian randomization methods, see Sheehan NA, Meng S, Didelez V. Mendelian randomisation: a tool for assessing causality in observational epidemiology. *Methods Mol Biol.* 2011;713:153–166.

Chapter 11. The Study of Mankind Is Man

Ibn Sina from the James Lind Library. The Library and Information Services Department of the the the Royal College of Physicians of Edinburgh. The James Lind Library website. http://www.jameslindlibrary.org/. Accessed April 20, 2011.

1. Penicillin was used to save the lives of countless wounded soldiers and civilians in World War II and became one of the most successful antibiotics ever discovered. Howard Florey was ennobled for his work by the queen of England and Anne Miller lived until the age of 90. In 1990, Oxford University awarded an honorary medical doctorate to Norman Heatley for his penicillin work, the first such degree ever awarded to a non-physician. Charles Florey, son of Howard, returned to Yale as a young academic and went on to a distinguished career as professor of epidemiology at Dundee. For more details on this episode, see Grossman CM. The first use of penicillin in the United States. *Ann Intern Med.* 2009;150(10):737; comment: *Ann Intern Med.* 2009;150(2):145–146; Norman Heatley obituary. *The Telegraph.* The Telegraph website. http://www.telegraph.co.uk/news/obituaries/1451046/ Norman-Heatley.html. January 7, 2004. Accessed April 26, 2012; Florey HW, Abraham EP. The work on penicillin at Oxford. *J Hist Med Allied Sci.* 1951;6(3):302–317.

2. Pope A. *An essay on man: poetical works.* Cary HF, ed. London: Routledge; 1870.

3. Pound P, Ebrahim S, Sandercock P, Bracken MB, Roberts I; Reviewing Animal Trials Systematically (RATS) Group: where is the evidence that animal research benefits humans? *BMJ.* 2004;328(7438):514–517.

4. Willett WC. The search for truth must go beyond statistics. *Epidemiology.* 2008; 19(5):655–656; discussion 657–658.

5. Ioannidis JP. Why most published research findings are false. *PLoS Med.* 2005; 2(8):e124.

6. Bracken MB. Why are so many epidemiology associations inflated or wrong? Does poorly conducted animal research suggest implausible hypotheses? *Ann Epidemiol.* 2009;19(3):220–224.

7. Stebbings R, Findlay L, Edwards C, et al. "Cytokine storm" in the phase 1 trial of monoclonal antibody TGN1412: better understanding the causes to improve preclinical testing of immunotherapeutics. *J Immunol.* 2007;179(5):3325–3331.

8. Corpet DE, Pierre F. How good are rodent models of carcinogenesis in predict-ing efficacy in humans? A systematic review and meta-analysis of colon chemo-prevention in rats, mice and men. *Eur J Cancer.* 2005;41(13):1911–1922; Corpet DE, Pierre F. Point: from animal models to prevention of colon cancer. Systematic review of chemoprevention in min mice and choice of the model system. *Cancer Epidemiol Biomarkers Prev.* 2003;12(5):391–400; Meister K, ed. *America's war on "carcinogens": reassessing the use of animal tests to predict human cancer risk.* American Council on Science and Health; 2005.

9. Pound P, Ebrahim S, Sandercock P, Bracken MB, Roberts I. Reviewing Animal Trials Systematically. Op. cit.

10. Macleod MR, O'Collins T, Horky LL, Howells DW, Donnan GA. Systematic review and metaanalysis of the efficacy of FK506 in experimental stroke. *J Cereb Blood Flow Metab.* 2005;25(6):713–721.

11. Mignini LE, Khan KS. Methodological quality of systematic reviews of animal studies: a survey of reviews of basic research. *BMC Med Res Methodol.* 2006;6:10.

12. Both quoted in Wade N. It may look authentic: here's how to tell it isn't. *New York Times.* New York Times website. http://www.nytimes.com/2006/01/24/science/24frau.html?_r=1&pagewanted=print. January 24, 2006. Accessed April 26, 2012.

13. Bracken MB. Why are so many epidemiology associations inflated or wrong? Op. cit.

14. Publication bias in animal research is a poorly studied phenomenon; four examples of investigations into it are: Neitzke U, Harder T, Schellong K, et al. Intrauterine growth restriction in a rodent model and developmental program-ming of the metabolic syndrome: a critical appraisal of the experimental evidence. *Placenta.* 2008;29(3):246–254; Macleod MR, O'Collins T, Howells DW, Donnan GA. Pooling of animal experimental data reveals influence of study design and publication bias. *Stroke.* 2004;35(5):1203–1208; Juutilainen J, Kumlin T, Naarala J. Do extremely low frequency magnetic fields enhance the effects of environ-mental carcinogens? A meta-analysis of experimental studies. *Int J Radiat Biol.* 2006;82(1):1–12; Dirx MJ, Zeegers MP, Dagnelie PC, van den Bogaard T, van den Brandt PA. Energy restriction and the risk of spontaneous mammary tumors in mice: a meta-analysis. *Int J Cancer.* 2003;106(5):766–770.

15. Perel P, Roberts I, Sena E, et al. Comparison of treatment effects between animal experiments and clinical trials: systematic review. *BMJ.* 2007;334 (7586):197.

16. Sena ES, Briscoe CL, Howells DW, Donnan GA, Sandercock PA, Macleod MR. Factors affecting the apparent efficacy and safety of tissue plasminogen activator in thrombotic occlusion models of stroke: systematic review and meta-analysis. *J Cereb Blood Flow Metab.* 2010;30(12):1905–1913.

17. Kilkenny C, Browne W, Cuthill IC, Emerson M, Altman DG. NC3Rs Reporting Guidelines Working Group. Animal research: reporting in vivo experiments: the ARRIVE guidelines. *Br J Pharmacol.* 2010;160(7):1577–1579.

18. Hooijmans C, de Vries R, Leenaars M, Ritskes-Hoitinga M. The Gold Standard Publication Checklist (GSPC) for improved design, reporting and scientific quality of animal studies GSPC versus ARRIVE guidelines. *Lab Anim.* 2011;45(1):61.

19. United States Environmental Protection Agency. *Guidelines for carcinogen risk sssessment.* United States Environmental Protection Agency: Washington, DC. EPA/630/R-00/004. September 24, 1986.

20. Knight A, Bailey J, Balcombe J. Animal carcinogenicity studies: 1. Poor human predictivity. *Altern Lab Anim.* 2006;34(1):19–27.

21. American Cancer Society website. *Known and probable human carcinogens.* http://www.cancer.org/Cancer/CancerCauses/OtherCarcinogens/General InformationaboutCarcinogens/known-and-probable-human-carcinogens. Last revised June 29, 2011. Accessed April 26, 2012.

22. Ibid.

23. Shanks N, Greek R, Greek J. Are animal models predictive for humans? *Philos Ethics Humanit Med.* 2009;4:2.

24. The Genetics Society of America. Spradling AC. *Learning the common language of genetics.* Genetics Society of America website. http://www.genetics.org/ content/174/1/1.long. 2006. Accessed April 26, 2012.

Chapter 12. Celebrity Trumps Science

1. Goldacre B. Bad science: fish oil exam results fail all the tests. *Guardian.* http://www.guardian.co.uk/commentisfree/2008/sep/27/medicalresearch. Published September 27, 2008. Accessed April 26, 2012; Goldacre B. Bad science: something fishy? *Guardian.* http://www.guardian.co.uk/science/2006/nov/11/badscience .uknews. Published November 10, 2006. Accessed April 26, 2012.

2. Rafii MS, Walsh S, Little JT, et al., and Alzheimer's Disease Cooperative Study. A phase II trial of huperzine A in mild to moderate Alzheimer disease. *Neurology.* 2011;76(16):1389–1394.

3. McCoy NL, Pitino L. Pheromonal influences on sociosexual behavior in young women. *Physiol Behav.* 2002;75(3):367–375; Cutler WB, Friedmann E, McCoy NL. Pheromonal influences on sociosexual behavior in men. *Arch Sex Behav.* 1998;27(1):1–13

4. Rokicki R. Advertising in the Roman Empire. *Whole Earth Review.* Spring 1987.

5. Food and Drug Administration. *Guidance for industry presenting risk information in prescription drug and medical device promotion,* May 2009.

6. Disclosure, I am a former trustee and sometime member of the board of directors of the American Council for Science and Health. Some of the material in this chapter is from *Celebrities vs. science.* American Council on Science and Health. New York; 2008.

7. Roberts L, Ahmed I, Hall S, Davison A. Intercessory prayer for the alleviation of ill health. *Cochrane Database Syst Rev.* 2009;(2):CD000368.

8. Dyer C. Wakefield was dishonest and irresponsible over MMR research, says GMC. *BMJ.* 2010;340:c593.

9. Institute of Medicine. *Adverse effects of vaccines: evidence and causality.* August 25, 2011.

10. Nattinger AB, Hoffmann RG, Howell-Pelz A, Goodwin JS. Effect of Nancy Reagan's mastectomy on choice of surgery for breast cancer by US women. *JAMA.* 1998;279(10):762–766.

11. Distefan JM, Pierce JP, Gilpin EA. Do favorite movie stars influence adolescent smoking initiation? *Am J Public Health.* 2004;94(7):1239–1244.

12. Brown WJ, Basil MD, Bocarnea MC. The influence of famous athletes on health beliefs and practices: Mark McGwire, child abuse prevention, and Androstenedione. *J Health Commun.* 2003;8(1):41–57.

13. Cheng AT, Hawton K, Lee CT, Chen TH. The influence of media reporting of the suicide of a celebrity on suicide rates: a population-based study. *Int J Epidemiol.* 2007;36(6):1229–1234.

Chapter 13. Replication and Pooling

1. Popper K. *Conjectures and refutations.* London: Routledge & K. Paul; 1963:33–39.

2. Clarke M, Chalmers I. Discussion sections in reports of controlled trials published in general medical journals: islands in search of continents? *JAMA.* 1998;280(3):280–282; Donne J. Meditation 17. In *Devotion upon emergent occasions;* 1623.

3. DeWan AT, Triche EW, Xu X, et al. PDE11A associations with asthma: results of a genome-wide association scan. *J Allergy Clin Immunol.* 2010;126(4): 871–873.e9.

4. Jüni P, Nartey L, Reichenbach S, Sterchi R, Dieppe PA, Egger M. Risk of cardiovascular events and rofecoxib: cumulative meta-analysis. *Lancet.* 2004; 364(9450):2021–2029. The Merck Pharmaceutical Company responded to the Jüni paper, claiming it had not included all the relevant trials.

5. Dr. William Black's work is cited in Tröhler, p. 117 (Tröhler U. *To improve the evidence of medicine: the 18th century British origins of a critical approach.* Edinburgh: Royal College of Physicians of Edinburgh; 2000); Prominent among the "arithmetic observationists" was John Haygarth who debunked the therapeutic value of Dr. Perkins's metallic tractors (see box 4.1).

6. Pearson K. Report on certain enteric fever inoculation statistics. *Br Med J.* 1904;2(2288):1243–1246. For more discussion of the history of systematic reviews, see Chalmers I, Hedges LV, Cooper H. A brief history of research synthesis. *Eval Health Prof.* 2002;25(1):12–37.

7. Goldberger J. Typhoid "bacillus carriers." In Rosenau MJ, Lumsden LL, Kastle JH. Report on the origin and prevalence of typhoid fever in the District of Columbia. *Hygienic Laboratory, Bulletin.* 1907;35:167–174. This work was first brought to my attention in Winkelstein W Jr. The first use of meta-analysis? *Am J Epidemiol.* 1998;147(8):717. More consideration of the early use of systematic reviews in epidemiology is in Bracken MB. Commentary: toward systematic reviews in epidemiology. *Int J Epidemiol.* 2001;30(5):954–957.

8. A. L. Cochrane obituary. *BMJ.* 1988;297:63.

9. Ibid.

10. Cochrane AL. 1931–1971: a critical review, with particular reference to the medical profession. In *Medicines for the year 2000.* London: Office of Health Economics; 1979;1–11.

11. Hetherington J, Dickersin K, Chalmers I, Meinert CL. Retrospective and prospective identification of unpublished controlled trials: lessons from a survey of obstetricians and pediatricians. *Pediatrics.* 1989;84(2):374–80.

12. Chalmers I, ed. Oxford database of perinatal trials. Oxford: Oxford University Press; 1988.

13. Chalmers I, Enkin M, Kierse M, eds. *Effective care in pregnancy and childbirth.* Oxford: Oxford University Press; 1989; Sinclair JC, Bracken MB, eds. *Effective care of the newborn infant.* Oxford: Oxford University Press; 1992.

14. A succinct history of the early years of the Cochrane Collaboration is available at Chalmers I, Sackett D, Silagy C. The Cochrane Collaboration. In Maynard A, Chalmers I, eds. *Non-random reflections on health services research.* London: BMJ Publishing Group; 1997:231–249. The longer-term impact of the Cochrane Collaboration is examined in Fox DM. Systematic reviews and health policy: the influence of a project on perinatal care since 1988. *Milbank Q.* 2011;89(3):425–449.

15. Chalmers I. The Cochrane Collaboration: preparing, maintaining and disseminating systematic reviews of the effects of health care. *Ann N Y Acad Sci.* 1993;703:

156–163. In Warren KS, Mosteller F, eds. *Doing more good than harm: the evaluation of health care interventions.* New York: New York Academy of Sciences; 1993.

16. Gøtzsche PC, Johansen HK. House dust mite control measures for asthma. *Cochrane Database Syst Rev.* 2008;(2):CD001187.

17. Garner SE, Fidan DD, Frankish R, Maxwell L. Rofecoxib for osteoarthritis. *Cochrane Database Syst Rev.* 2005;(1):CD005115.

18. Horton R. Vioxx, the implosion of Merck, and aftershocks at the FDA. *Lancet.* 2004;364(9450):1995–1996.

19. Bracken MB. Oral contraception and congenital malformations in offspring: a review and meta-analysis of the prospective studies. *Obstet Gynecol.* 1990;76(3 Pt 2):552–557.

20. Crowley P, Chalmers I, Keirse MJ. The effects of corticosteroid administration before preterm delivery: an overview of the evidence from controlled trials. *Br J Obstet Gynaecol.* 1990;97(1):11–25.

21. Sinclair JC. Meta-analysis of randomized controlled trials of antenatal corticosteroid for the prevention of respiratory distress syndrome: discussion. *Am J Obstet Gynecol.* 1995;173(1):335–344.

22. Chalmers I. Electronic publications for updating controlled trial reviews. *Lancet.* 1986;2(8501):287.

23. Chalmers I, ed. Oxford database of perinatal trials. Oxford: Oxford University Press; 1988.

24. Lau J, Antman EM, Jimenez-Silva J, Kupelnick B, Mosteller F, Chalmers TC. Cumulative meta-analysis of therapeutic trials for myocardial infarction. *N Engl J Med.* 1992;327(4):248–254.

25. Clarke M, Stewart L, Pignon JP, Bijnens L. Individual patient data meta-analysis in cancer. *Br J Cancer.* 1998;77(11):2036–2044.

26. Effects of adjuvant tamoxifen and of cytotoxic therapy on mortality in early breast cancer. An overview of 61 randomized trials among 28,896 women. Early Breast Cancer Trialists' Collaborative Group. *N Engl J Med.* 1988;319(26):1681–1692; Ovarian ablation in early breast cancer: overview of the randomised trials. Early Breast Cancer Trialists' Collaborative Group. *Lancet.* 1996;348(9036):1189–1196.

27. McLernon DJ, Harrild K, Bergh C, et al. Clinical effectiveness of elective single versus double embryo transfer: meta-analysis of individual patient data from randomised trials. *BMJ.* 2010;341:c6945.

Chapter 14. Bias in Publication and Reporting

1. Hopkins issues internal review committee report on research volunteer's death. Johns Hopkins Medicine website. http://www.hopkinsmedicine.org/press/2001/JULY/010716.htm. July 16, 2001. Accessed April 26, 2012.

2. Other searches in PubMed do produce a large literature on hexamethonium. Searched May 29, 2011. MEDLINE is the database published by the National Library of Medicine; PubMed is the part of it typically used to search the literature because it includes journal articles before they have been formally published in a print journal. MEDLINE has highly sophisticated technical strategies for indexing articles to help searching. As of May 2011, it included over 20 million articles in the biomedical and life sciences literature and electronic books.

3. Turner EH, Matthews AM, Linardatos E, Tell RA, Rosenthal R. Selective publication of antidepressant trials and its influence on apparent efficacy. *N Engl J Med.* 2008;358(3):252–260.

4. Dickersin K, Min YI, Meinert CL. Factors influencing publication of research results: follow-up of applications submitted to two institutional review boards. *JAMA.* 1992;267(3):374–378.

5. Blumenthal D, Campbell EG, Anderson MS, Causino N, Louis KS. Withholding research results in academic life science: evidence from a national survey of faculty. *JAMA.* 1997;277(15):1224–1228. 410 per 2,167 (19.8 percent) US life science faculty responding to a 1995 survey reported delaying publication beyond six months.

6. Easterbrook PJ, Berlin JA, Gopalan R, Matthews DR. Publication bias in clinical research. *Lancet.* 1991;337(8746):867–872; Hopewell S, Clarke M, Stewart L, Tierney J. Time to publication for results of clinical trials. *Cochrane Database Syst Rev.* 2007;(2):MR000011.

7. Ioannidis JP. Effect of the statistical significance of results on the time to completion and publication of randomized efficacy trials. *JAMA.* 1998;279(4): 281–286.

8. Stern JM, Simes RJ. Publication bias: evidence of delayed publication in a cohort study of clinical research projects. *BMJ.* 1997;315(7109):640–645.

9. Hopewell S, Clarke M, Lefebvre C, Scherer R. Hand searching versus electronic searching to identify reports of randomized trials. *Cochrane Database Syst Rev* 2007;(2):MR000001.

10. Illuzzi JL, Bracken MB. Duration of intrapartum prophylaxis for neonatal Group B streptococcal disease: a systematic review. *Obstet Gynecol.* 2006; 108(5):1254–1265.

11. Chan AW, Hróbjartsson A, Haahr MT, Gøtzsche PC, Altman DG. Empirical evidence for selective reporting of outcomes in randomized trials: comparison of protocols to published articles. *JAMA.* 2004;291(20):2457–2465.

12. Ibid.

13. Gould SJ. *The structure of evolutionary theory.* Cambridge: Harvard University Press; 2002:763–764.

14. Turner EH, Matthews AM, Linardatos E, Tell RA, Rosenthal R. Selective publication of antidepressant trials. Op. cit.

15. Petitjean ME, Pointillart V, Dixmerias F, et al. Traitement medicamenteux de la lesion medullaire traumatique au stade aigu. *Ann Fr Anesth Reanim.* 1998;17(2):114–122; Pointillart V, Petitjean ME, Wiart L, et al. Pharmacological therapy of spinal cord injury during the acute phase. *Spinal Cord.* 2000;38(2):71–76.

16. Errami M, Hicks JM, Fisher W, et al. Déjà vu–a study of duplicate citations in Medline. *Bioinformatics.* 2008;24(2):243–249.

17. The most recent paper in the series at time of writing is Vajda FJ, Graham J, Hitchcock AA, O'Brien TJ, Lander CM, Eadie MJ. Foetal malformations after exposure to antiepileptic drugs in utero assessed at birth and 12 months later: observations from the Australian pregnancy register. *Acta Neurol Scand.* 2011;124(1):9–12.

18. The most recent paper is Reis M, Källén B. Delivery outcome after maternal use of antidepressant drugs in pregnancy: an update using Swedish data. *Psychol Med.* 2010;40(10):1723–1733.

19. Louik C, Lin AE, Werler MM, Hernández-Díaz S, Mitchell AA. First-trimester use of selective serotonin-reuptake inhibitors and the risk of birth defects. *N Engl J Med.* 2007;356(26):2675–2683, and Alwan S, Reefhuis J, Rasmussen SA, Olney RS, Friedman JM; National Birth Defects Prevention Study. Use of selective serotonin-reuptake inhibitors in pregnancy and the risk of birth defects. *N Engl J Med.* 2007;356(26):2684–2692.

20. Ibid.

21. Dickersin K, Min YI, Meinert CL. Factors influencing publication of research results. Op. cit.

22. Bracken MB. Preregistration of epidemiology protocols: a commentary in support. *Epidemiology.* 2011;22(2):135–137.

Chapter 15. Causes

1. Ferguson N. *Empire: how Britain made the modern world.* New York: Penguin Books; 2004:185.

2. Leistner M. The Times Beach story. Synthesis/Regeneration website. www.greens .org/s-r/078/07–09.html. Summer 1995. Accessed April 26, 2012.

3. US Environmental Protection Agency. Joint federal/state action taken to relocate Times Beach residents (EPA press release, February 22, 1983). Environmental Protection Agency website. www.epa.gov/history/topics/times/02.html. Last updated June 8, 2011. Accessed April 26, 2012.

4. Institute of Medicine. *Veterans and Agent Orange: update 2006.* Institute of Medicine website. http://www.iom.edu/Reports/2007/Veterans-and-Agent-Orange-Update-2006.aspx Last updated August 17, 2011. Accessed April 26, 2012.

5. Institute of Medicine. *Veterans and Agent Orange: update 2008.* Institute of Medicine website. http://www.iom.edu/Reports/2009/Veterans-and-Agent-Orange-Update-2008.aspx. Last updated August 17, 2011. Accessed April 26, 2012.

6. Starr TB. Significant issues raised by meta-analyses of cancer mortality and dioxin exposure. *Environ Health Perspect.* 2003;111(12):1443–1447.

7. Taussig HB. A study of the German outbreak of phocomelia: the thalidomide syndrome. *JAMA.* 1962;180:1106–1114.

8. Hill AB. The environment and disease: association or causation? *Proc R Soc Med.* 1965;58:295–300.

9. Rothman KJ, Greenland S, Lash TL. *Modern epidemiology.* 3rd ed. Philadelphia: Wolters Kluwer / Lippincott Williams & Wilkins; 2008:30.

10. Bradford Hill was also the leading medical statistician of his generation, and he made other notable observations concerning the use of statistical tests and statistical significance that are discussed in chapter 8.

11. Barton A. Chapter 25: Causation. In Powers M, Harris N, Barton A, eds. *Clinical negligence.* 4th ed. Edinburgh: Tottel Publishing; 2008.

12. Ibid.

13. *Daubert v Merrell Dow Pharmaceuticals Inc.*, 113 S. Ct. 2786 (1993).

14. The original paper is Jick H, Watkins RN, Hunter JR, et al. Replacement estrogens and endometrial cancer. *N Engl J Med.* 1979;300(5):218–222. The critical but flawed comparison: Horwitz RI, Feinstein AR, Horwitz SM, Robboy SJ. Necropsy diagnosis of endometrial cancer and detection-bias in case/control studies. *Lancet.* 1981;2(8237):66–68.

15. Klein RJ, Zeiss C, Chew EY, et al. Complement factor H polymorphism in age-related macular degeneration. *Science.* 2005;308(5720):385–389; Marcos M, Gómez-Munuera M, Pastor I, González-Sarmiento R, Laso FJ. Tumor necrosis factor polymorphisms and alcoholic liver disease: a HuGE review and meta-analysis. *Am J Epidemiol.* 2009;170(8):948–956.

16. Susser M. What is a cause and how do we know one? A grammar for pragmatic epidemiology. *Am J Epidemiol.* 1991;133(7):635–648.

17. Ford D, Easton DF, Stratton M, et al. Genetic heterogeneity and penetrance analysis of the BRCA1 and BRCA2 genes in breast cancer families. The Breast Cancer Linkage Consortium. *Am J Hum Genet.* 1998;62(3):676–689.

18. Barnhart HX, Caldwell B, Thomas B, et al. Natural history of human immunodeficiency virus disease in perinatally infected children: an analysis from the Pediatric Spectrum of Disease Project. *Pediatrics.* 1996;97(5):710–716.

Chapter 16. Ultimate Causation

Simon Hoggart of the *Guardian* reported the mustard label. There were several other warning labels, including one that came with a Philips television set cautioning not to "kick it, hit it with a hammer, or set fire to it."

1. There is debate as to when the pump handle was removed after Snow documented that this particular supply of water was associated with increased cholera risk. It

also seems possible that the cholera epidemic was declining before the pump handle was removed. Nonetheless, this iconic moment in the history of epidemiology is properly celebrated as a triumph of observational epidemiology.

2. Green J, Cairns BJ, Casabonne D, Wright FL, Reeves G, Beral V; Million Women Study collaborators. Height and cancer incidence in the Million Women Study: prospective cohort, and meta-analysis of prospective studies of height and total cancer risk. *Lancet Oncol.* 2011;12(8):785–794.

3. Aristotle. *Physics.* 11. 9.200b 4–7.

4. Hecht SS. Cigarette smoking and lung cancer: chemical mechanisms and approaches to prevention. *Lancet Oncol.* 2002;3(8):461–469.

5. Hanahan D, Weinberg RA. Hallmarks of cancer: the next generation. *Cell.* 2011; 144(5):646–674.

6. At the time of this writing there is no compelling evidence for any increased risk of cancer being associated with cell phone use.

7. Krieger N. Epidemiology and the web of causation: has anyone seen the spider? *Soc Sci Med.* 1994;39(7):887–903.

8. Ng SF, Lin RC, Laybutt DR, Barres R, Owens JA, Morris MJ. Chronic high-fat diet in fathers programs β-cell dysfunction in female rat offspring. *Nature.* 2010; 467(7318):963–966.

9. Bracken MB, Belanger K, Cookson WO, Triche E, Christiani DC, Leaderer BP. Genetic and perinatal risk factors for asthma onset and severity: a review and theoretical analysis. *Epidemiol Rev.* 2002;24(2):176–189.

10. Hopefully, art gallery and museum curators will not object to their noun being coopted, but "curation" is a convenient term to emphasize how causation, the origins of disease, and curation, treating disease, are analogous constructs when one considers how data supporting each of them should be examined for evidence of study validity.

11. Sigma 2 is actually 0.954 or 1 in 22, R. A. Fisher rounded to 5 percent or 1 in 20 for simplicity. Also see chapter 8.

12. For an insightful analysis see "Nuclear energy" in Lovelock J. *The vanishing face of Gaia: a final warning.* New York: Basic Books; 2009:105.

Alexander FE, Boyle P, eds. *Methods for investigating localized clustering of disease.* IARC Scientific Publications No. 135. Lyon, France: IARC; 1996.

Blastland M, Dilnot A. *The tiger that isn't: seeing through a world of numbers.* London: Profile Books; 2007.

Chalmers I, Enkin M, Keirse MJNC, eds. *Effective care in pregnancy and childbirth.* Oxford: Oxford University Press; 1989.

Cochrane AL. *Effectiveness and efficiency: random reflections on health services.* London: Nuffield Provincial Hospitals Trust; 1972.

Collins HM. *Changing order: replication and induction in scientific practice.* Chicago: University of Chicago Press; 1985.

Cooper H, Hedges LV, Valentine SC. *The handbook of research synthesis and meta-analysis.* 2nd ed. New York: Russell Sage Foundation; 2009.

Dawkins R. *The greatest show on earth: the evidence for evolution.* London: Bantam Press; 2009.

Entine J. *Scared to death: how chemophobia threatens public health.* New York: American Council on Science and Health; 2011.

Fuller JG. *Fever! The hunt for a new killer virus.* New York: Readers Digest Press; 1974.

Garrett L. *The coming plague: newly emerging diseases in a world out of balance.* New York: Penguin Books; 1995.

Goldacre B. *Bad science.* London: Fourth Estate; 2008.

Greene B. *The hidden reality: parallel universes and the deep laws of the cosmos.* London: Allen Lane; 2011.

Hardy A. *The epidemic streets: infectious disease and the rise of preventive medicine, 1856–1900.* Oxford: Clarendon Press; 1993.

Illich I. *Medical nemesis: the expropriation of health.* London: Calder & Boyers; 1975.

Irwig L, Irwig J, Trevena L, Sweet M. *Smart health choices: making sense of health advice.* London: Hammersmith Press, 2007.

Johnson S. *The ghost map: the story of London's most terrifying epidemic--and how it changed science, cities, and the modern world.* New York: Riverhead Books; 2006.

Kahneman D. *Thinking, fast and slow.* New York: Farrar, Straus and Giroux; 2011.

Keating C. *Smoking kills: the revolutionary life of Richard Doll.* Oxford: Signal Books; 2009.

Law S. *Believing bullshit: how not to get sucked into an intellectual black hole.* Amherst, NY: Promethius Books; 2011.

Lax E. *The mold in Dr. Florey's coat.* New York: Henry Holt; 2004

Maynard A, Chalmers I, eds. *Non-random reflections on health services research: on the 25th anniversary of Archie Cochrane's Effectiveness and Efficiency.* London: BMJ Publishing; 1997.

Mnookin S. *The panic virus: a true story of medicine, science and fear.* New York: Simon and Schuster; 2011.

Monot J. Wainhouse A, trans. *Chance and necessity: an essay on the natural philosophy of modern biology.* New York: Vintage Books; 1972. First published as *"Le hazard et la nécessité."* Éditions du Seuil; 1970.

Offit PA. *Deadly choices: how the anti-vaccine movement threatens us all.* Philadelphia: Basic Books; 2011.

Popper KR. *Objective knowledge.* Oxford: Clarendon Press; 1972.

Rothman KR, ed. *Causal inference.* Chestnut Hill, MA: Epidemiology Resources; 1988.

Silverman WA. *Human experimentation: a guided step into the unknown.* Oxford: Oxford University Press; 1985.

——. *Where's the evidence? debates in modern medicine.* Oxford: Oxford University Press; 1998.

Sinclair JC, Bracken MB, eds. *Effective care of the newborn infant.* Oxford: Oxford University Press; 1992.

Susser M. *Causal thinking in the health sciences: concepts and strategies in epidemiology.* New York: Oxford University Press; 1973.

Terris M, ed. *Goldberger on pellagra.* Baton Rouge: Louisiana State University; 1964.

Tröhler U. *To improve the evidence of medicine: the 18th century British origins of a critical approach.* Edinburgh: Royal College of Physicians of Edinburgh; 2000.

Woloshin S, Schwartz LM, Welch G. *Know your chances: understanding health statistics.* Berkeley: University of California Press; 2008.

Woolfson A. *An intelligent person's guide to genetics.* New York: Overlook Press; 2004.

Babies. *See* Preterm babies and lung problems
Babylonians, 54
Bachmann, Michele, 197–98
Baigent, Colin, 70, 75
Barton, Anthony, 248–49
Bartter syndrome, 161
Bayes, Thomas, 289n8
Bayesian approach to probability, 136, 289n8
Bell curve (normal distribution), 131–32, 139–40, 274. *See also* Statistical analysis
Bell's palsy, 194
Ben Cao Tu Jing, 53
Bendectin, 21–23, 248, 249
Benzene, 175, 263
Beriberi, 7
Beta carotene supplementation, 78, 268, 275
Bhopal, India, gas leak, 146–47
Bias: ascertainment of exposure bias, 92; and choice of comparator, 104–6; confounding and residual confounding, 89, 99–103; correlation versus causation, 107–12; definition of, 88, 281n1; dependent observation bias, 98–99; diagnostic test bias, 122–23; disease ascertainment bias, 91–92; duplicitous and duplicate publication, 234–37; file drawer bias, 225–26; indication bias, 49, 96–97; language bias, 212; lead-time screening bias, 120, 121; length-time screening bias, 120, 121; and lumping or splitting disease diagnoses, 106–7; multiple comparison bias, 49, 64–65, 97–98, 286n11; outcome reporting bias, 232–34; prognostic-test bias, 123–25;

"protopathic" (early disease) bias, 104; publication bias, 49, 51, 178–79, 224–38, 248, 293n14; recall bias, 92–95; reverse causality, 49, 103–4; screening test bias, 120, 121; selection bias, 89–91; sources and types of, 49, 89–112, 285n4; stage migration bias, 124–25; underestimation of, 51; and very, very large observational studies, 110
Biological plausibility, 177, 202, 246
Biology, 33, 183–84, 191
Bipolar disorder, 159
Birth control. *See* Contraceptives
Birth defects: in animals, 175, and antidepressants during pregnancy, 91–92, 236–37; and antiepileptic drugs during pregnancy, 39–40, 96, 105, 202, 235–36; and antinausea drug during pregnancy, 21–23, 98–99; genetic component of, 20, 157; heart malformations, 31, 91, 106–7; National Birth Defects Prevention Study, 107; oral contraceptive exposure in pregnancy and limb reduction defects, 217, 218; and paroxetine (Paxil) during pregnancy, 237; registries recording, 90, 235–37; and sodium valproate during pregnancy, 22, 39–40, 251–52; and thalidomide during pregnancy, 41, 175, 242–43, 247, 251–52, 264, 281n10. *See also* Teratogens and teratogenesis
Bisphenol-A (BPA), 255, 276
Bisphosphonates, 179
Black, William, 204
"Black box," 264
Black Death, 162. *See also* Bubonic plague